EXPLORING CAREERS IN DENTISTRY

By

Jessica A. Rickert, D.D.S.

THE ROSEN PUBLISHING GROUP, INC.

New York

This book has been updated to include
the latest available statistics.

Published in 1983, 1985, 1988, 1991 by The Rosen Publishing Group, Inc.
29 East 21st Street, New York, NY 10010

Copyright 1983, 1985, 1988, 1991 by   Jessica A. Rickert

Revised Edition 1991

Library of Congress Cataloging-in-Publication Data
Rickert, Jessica A.
  Exploring careers in dentistry.

Includes glossary and index.
  (Exploring careers)
  Summary: Discusses the profession of dentistry and
offers advice to those interested in dentistry as a
career.
  1. Dentistry—Vocational guidance—Juvenile literature.
[1. Dentistry—Vocational guidance. 2. Vocational
guidance] I. Title. II. Series: Exploring careers
(Rosen Publishing Group)
RK60.R5 1983   617.6′023   83-8673
ISBN 0-8239-1373-2

Manufactured in the United States of America

Contents

About the Author

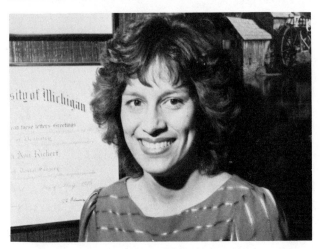

Jessica A. Rickert, D.D.S. (William A. Strait Photography).

Jessica A. Rickert, D.D.S., is a graduate of the University of Michigan School of Dentistry. She has been in private practice for eight years. For five years she was the director of the Dental Clinic at the Children's Aid Society, a private agency for foster-care children in the Detroit area; there, she initiated programs in preventive dentistry and orthodontia. She has served on the Michigan Urban Indian Health Council, and she helped found a dental clinic at the Detroit Urban Indian Health Clinic.

She is active in the American Dental Association, having chaired the Oakland County Dental Society's Speakers' Bureau; she also serves on the Michigan Dental Association's Public Relations Committee.

She and her husband, William A. Strait, have three children: Carole, Tom, and Brandon. Dr. Rickert has enjoyed serving on the Parent–Teacher–Student Association, in the Girl Scouts of America, and as a coach in girls' sports. She also is a member of the Chamber of Commerce.

I

All of us girls were standing around the halls after school. We were so nervous, trying out for the spring musical. I have a pretty good voice, and I hoped to get a part, maybe even the LEAD.

About a year and a half ago, I never would have thought of doing this. I mostly sat at home, watching TV or doing crosswords. Mom and Dad were always on my case to get out and do things, but I was just too embarrassed. Ever since I could remember, I had been in speech therapy because of a silly lisp. Besides, my smile was awful looking. I rarely smiled or laughed because I didn't want the kids to see my teeth; the upper ones were way up under my lip, and they jutted forward. I asked Dad about braces, but he said they were pretty expensive and we couldn't afford them right now.

Mom went to a new dentist for a filling and told her about my problem. Dr. White said to bring me in and she'd take a look.

It turned out to be a "tongue-thrust habit" that was causing my whole problem. Dr. White took an impression of my mouth with some gooey stuff and fitted me with a wire that kept my tongue away from my upper teeth when I swallowed. It was pretty hard to do at first, and a couple of times food or water spewed out from between my lips.

Dr. White had me practice saying "fifty-five" and "sixty-six" and "Mississippi" over and over again, showing me

1

where my tongue and lips were supposed to be. Then she had me promise to read one chapter a night out loud, in my bedroom, from a book she lent me. She said that in a little while my lisp would go away.

Dad said the wire cost about one-twentieth what regular braces would. And, just as Dr. White said, my top teeth moved down and back, like a garage door closing, as I did the exercises she had shown me. I had to wear the wire for a full year.

When the school announced try-outs for the spring play, Mom encouraged me to go ahead and try out. I can't believe I'm doing it, but I don't have to worry about my teeth any more, or that ridiculous lisp.

When I grow up, I think I'll be a dentist just like Dr. White and help someone else with their teeth.

This is Heather Oakland's story. She is an eighth-grader at Washington Junior High School. And she did get a part in the school musical.

Chapter I

Nature of the Profession

A dentist has a Doctorate of Dental Surgery or a Doctorate of Medical Dentistry; both are equivalent degrees. This doctor is responsible for the health of the lower one-third of the patient's face—the underlying bone structure, the overlying muscles and skin, the soft tissues inside the mouth, the hidden nerves and glands, and, of course, the teeth themselves and their supporting structures. Without the satisfactory health, form, and function of the lower one-third of our faces, we would have difficulty speaking, expressing emotion, and eating.

What is health? As defined by the World Health Organization, "Health is a state of complete physical, mental, and social well-being, and not merely the absence of disease." Can every person obtain health? How can the dentist help the patient?

Who is the dentist? He or she is a recognized expert, an educated doctor whose talents and skills and judgment are sought after and respected. This special person is expected to serve humanity to the best of his or her ability; the individual patient expects the dentist to keep this promise. The unique doctor-patient relationship from ancient times has been built upon the most idealistic of human values, and the dentist must never forget this pledge.

Who is the patient? The patient is you and I and every other human being we've ever seen. They are young, attractive, and happy. They are old and gloomy. They are rich and sophisticated; sometimes they are poor and lazy. The mayor or governor may walk into the dentist's office with a problem. So might a parolee. A two-year-old toddler might come in with a fractured front tooth; so might a magazine model; so might a fellow who tripped in the middle of his tennis game, smelly and sweaty; so might a great-great grandma, with a broken denture tooth. The dentist must treat all these people with the same dedication to excellence. The dentist's basic love for humanity—all of humanity—cannot waver, and it will not change if the dentist can remind him or herself of the Patient's Bill of Rights.[1] After all, the dentist will also be a patient some day:

1. The patient has the right to considerate and respectful care.
2. The patient has the right to obtain from the dentist complete current information regarding his diagnosis, treatment, and prognosis in terms the patient can reasonably be expected to understand.
3. The patient has the right to receive from his dentist information necessary to give informed consent prior to the start of any procedure or treatment. Where a dentally significant alternative for care exists, or when the patient requests information concerning alternatives, the patient has the right to such information.
4. The patient has the right to refuse treatment to the extent permitted by law, and to be informed of the consequences of his action.
5. The patient has the right to every consideration of his privacy concerning his own dental care program.
6. The patient has the right to expect that all communi-

---

[1] Adapted, with permission, from *Patient's Bill of Rights, published by the American Hospital Association,* © 1975.

cations and records pertaining to his care should be treated as confidential.

7. The patient has the right to request that within its capacity a dental facility must make a reasonable response to the request of a patient for services.
8. The patient has the right to be advised as to the untested, possibly experimental, treatment affecting his care . . . and the right to refuse such care.
9. The patient has the right to expect reasonable continuity of care.
10. The patient has the right to examine and receive an explanation of his bill regardless of the source of payment.
11. The patient has the right to know what rules apply to his conduct as a patient in a dental facility.

Anyone considering dentistry as a career must realize that he or she will have to integrate many diverse factors in determining and delivering optimal care. The dentist also

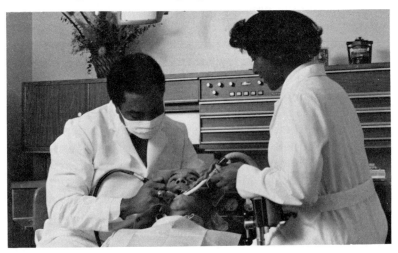

Dr. James Wright offers his patients the latest in dental science and technology in his modern office in Pontiac, Michigan.

has to balance various facets of professional life and personal life. He or she must be empathetic and compassionate, but also reasonable and intelligent. He or she must be decisive and self-motivated, but also nonjudgmental and understanding. Most dentists are found to be individualistic and independent; nevertheless, the dentist is part of a team and must operate in cooperation with the office personnel, other dentists and specialists, and other health professionals. The required persistence and dedication to technical excellence must be weighed against reasonable human expectations and performance. These multifaceted decisions make up a dentist's everyday existence. All this does produce stress and strain for any dentist; but even then, the dentist cannot give up until the patient is adequately cared for. Although dentistry is plain hard work, the satisfaction of a successful course of treatment is emotionally and intellectually satisfying.

Any patient may exhibit an affliction and the dentist is expected to possess the knowledge and the ability to remedy the immediate situation. What kinds of abnormalities are we talking about?

The most common problem is the caries process, "cavities." These are caused by bacteria, *Streptococcus mutans*, that are found in everyone's mouth except those of newborn babies or persons sealed in sterile environments. Dental science leads us to believe that all caries are preventable, but human beings and their habits have not responded to those scientific findings yet. Another common disease is periodontitis, or "gum disease." Various types are described in the dental literature, but common to all types is the accumulation of plaque and calculus and several types of bacteria along the gumline. This focus of irritation is like a sliver underneath the cuticle of a fingernail; eventually the inflammation causes the tissue to pull away, and the tooth becomes loose. This disease is also preventable and reversible if detected and treated at an early stage; again, the patient's cooperation is required.

There are degenerative changes that can affect the facial muscles, even paralyze these muscles. Often, the dentist is the first medical person consulted about vague, tingly sensations that may precede conditions such as palsies and tics. The dentist has to rule out any local contributing factor such as an infected wisdom tooth before referring the patient to a neurologist. The tongue, also, can mirror a patient's underlying health according to its color, texture, and consistency. Its very structure can cause speech problems for youngsters, and its alteration, intentional or otherwise, can handicap adults. In fact, dentists have to be knowledgeable about speech development and may have to engage in some speech therapy.

Developmental abnormalities and injury of the hard and soft palates are approached by a team of dental specialists, including the general practitioner. The underlying bony structures of the lower face include the tempromandibular joint and ligaments, the mandible and maxilla, the floors of the nose and sinus cavities, and the palate. The strength and integrity of these bones can be severely compromised by abcesses, cysts, and trauma. Very often, a traumatized patient may be unaware of damage more significant than an avulsed (knocked out) tooth; the dentist's exam or X rays may very well reveal jaw fractures or torn muscles. Because of prompt referral, the patient can be returned to optimal health.

The dentist is also responsible for the primary detection of lesions suggestive of oral cancer. After treatment, patients with cancer of the head and neck are extremely susceptible to caries and periodontitis, and their oral condition has to be handled with the utmost care. Although such a patient is referred to a medical complex, the dentist is often the primary diagnostician and so becomes an important support person upon the patient's return to daily life.

Infectious diseases such as herpes and even chicken pox can manifest themselves primarily in the oral cavity; or, like hepatitis and tuberculosis, can be readily transmitted by the saliva and blood. The dentist is obligated to protect not only him or herself and the office personnel, but also the public at large, from transmission of these diseases.

There are many sociological and psychological ills the dentist must be aware of and guard against. He or she is obligated by law to report suspected cases of child abuse and may even have to testify in court about such cases. Forensic medicine includes forensic dentistry, and a dentist or his or her records may identify a corpse. Drug abuse is found everywhere, and the dentist has to be wary of addicts attempting to procure drugs through faked oral illness. It is the dentist's personal responsibility to strive to make sure these drugs are safely used for the treatment of the diseases they were developed for when he or she puts the pen to the prescription pad.

The dentists cannot numerically provide every phase of treatment for all their patients, and so they must work

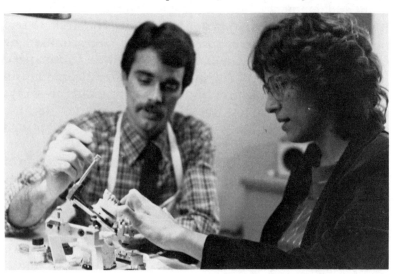

Dr. Jessica Rickert discusses a difficult case with laboratory technician, D.H. Baker. They are using a Denar Articulator to simulate jaw movements (William A. Strait Photography).

within a team. These are the dental personnel who must be supervised on a daily basis, including the registered dental hygienist, the dental assistant, the business personnel, and the dental laboratory technician. Although any of these auxiliaries may be providing an actual phase of treatment for a patient, the dentist is ultimately responsible for any action and its outcome to a patient for care received under his or her direction.

The general dentist also must coordinate his or her efforts with a host of dental and medical specialists. A teenager may be seeing a general dentist for caries control, an orthodontist for braces, and an oral surgeon for extractions. All three professionals must cooperate closely and be in communication as to the various phases of treatment in order for all treatments to culminate successfully. The general dentist is the most likely source of referral to the numerous specialists. He or she must maintain contact with the other doctors and must be convinced that the specialist he or she has referred a patient to is a capable and competent practitioner.

The dentist can never slack off or take the easy way out, regardless of his or her personal feelings or situation. Continuity of care for the patients must be established before the dentist becomes unable to render care. The responsibility of every practitioner in a medical field cannot be overemphasized. At the same time, the joy and fulfillment a successful practitioner achieves are extremely rewarding and satisfying. Obviously, dentistry is not a wise career choice unless a person is absolutely certain he or she can shoulder the responsibility and will make the sacrifices required as well as enjoy the benefits.

II

My dentist was getting older, so he decided to retire, and a nice young fellow took over his practice. I was due for a checkup, and this young fellow, Dr. Muratore, informed me that it was time for a new set of X rays. I gave him a hard time at first, because it seems as if all these young doctors, not just dentists, are always trying to X-ray everybody. Finally, he convinced me that it was necessary.

It's a good thing I let him do it, because a strange thing showed up on the film. In my lower right jaw was an odd-looking conglomeration of "radiopacity." The doctor said it was some kind of tumor with a fancy name. I just wanted to know if it was cancer. He said the only way to find out was to have it biopsied, but that usually these types of tumors were benign. I was referred to a Dr. Largot, an oral surgeon.

Dr. Largot advised me to have the whole thing out, in the hospital. He said it was good that the growth was discovered at this early stage, because any tumor, cancerous or not, can hollow out the jawbone and seriously endanger the jaw and its teeth. I was admitted to the hospital the following Wednesday and had the operation on Thursday. Luckily, it was benign! I was so happy that I wanted to dance. I left the hospital on Saturday, with a sore mouth and a glad heart.

I know Dr. Muratore got a report from the oral surgeon, but I never told him how grateful I am to him for insisting on the X rays and for the prompt referral. Yep, Dr. Muratore is one smart cookie.

This is the story of forty-five-year-old Donald Martell. Mr. Martell is tandem truck driver whose wife had to force him to go to the dentist for checkups because he "was always too dad-burned busy to be bothered." Now he never misses an appointment and is always referring new patients to Dr. Muratore.

Chapter II

Dentists at Work

In what kind of environment will a dentist spend his or her day? It is most probable that he or she will occupy a variation of the basic medical/dental office arrangement in a professional building. The dentist will be indoors all day, and the majority of time will be spent in an operatory. These may be small rooms arranged in a row; or an open layout may be used, with the chairs arranged in a circle and a short partition between them. The operatory itself is small, because of the proximity of the dentist to the patient, the equipment, and the dental assistant. The dentist is seldom more than twelve inches away from the patient; in fact, the dentist is necessarily in very close proximity to the patient's face. One fellow even observed that the intimacy between the dentist and the patient is only surpassed by that between husband and wife! This constant nearness is noticed by every patient a dentist treats, and is remembered. Being "on stage" all day long can be tiring to the dentist, and he or she has to guard against becoming "peopled out."

Virtually all dentists and assistants now operate sitting down, near the patient's shoulder or behind the patient. Basically, the requirements are: the patient's chair, an assistant's stool, the dentist's chair, a cabinet, an X-ray machine, and the dental unit and light. The dental unit provides the power for the handpieces and other instruments. In addition to the operatory, there is a reception room with adequate seating and furnishings to make the patients comfortable. A business office is essential. A dental laboratory and a darkroom must be included, as well as a bathroom. To this minimal setup, many dentists prefer to add a number of operatories, a private office, an employee's lounge, and a storage room.

Even in clinic situations, the dentist can expect to find these basic features in the dental area; a difference, though, is that he or she will be close to other medical specialty treatment areas such as pediatric examining rooms or medical laboratories. The reception room, business office, and bathroom will likely be shared with the other medical personnel. Many government or private programs include mobile dental equipment. This may be permanently installed in a bus or van; or the apparatus may be packed in cases, necessitating assembly and an electrical supply before patients can be treated.

Private practitioners can modify their offices to suit their own style. One dentist loved cowboys and so he decorated his office and operatories to look like a Western town of old. Another man installed a swimming pool in his reception room for patients, personnel, and family use. Another designed his office like a futuristic spaceship, even to the point of having all the personnel wear spacesuit-like uniforms. A woman dentist used the idea of a French garden, with plants and statues and water fountains set off against wall murals of foliage; natural light flooded in through many skylights. Some dentists use their offices to show off talents in other areas; an amateur photographer has a captive audience for his personal "photo gallery," a weaver can use her creations to soften her rooms, a potter can display his ceramic creations, and a woodworker can even build some of the furniture in the office. It's easy to see that, although there are physical restrictions, a private doctor can be as conservative or imaginative as he or she desires in decorating the dental office.

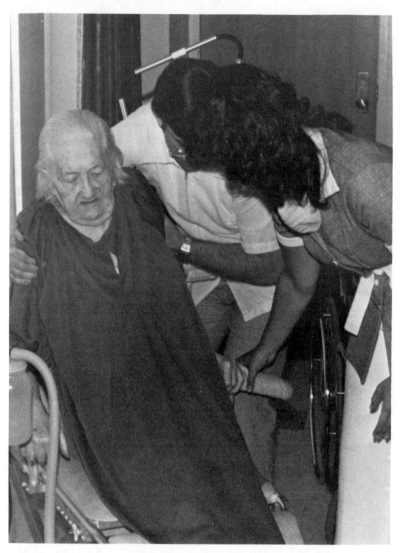

A dentist and a hygienist from the Tri-County Dental Health Council help a geriatric patient into the dental chair. The Council has a mobile dental chair, unit, light, air compressor, and X-ray machine. All the apparatus is contained in four "footlockers" and can be transported and used wherever there is electric power and water.

The dentist also has the privilege of practicing anywhere in the country he or she has obtained a license. There is no national license for dentists, and usually the dentist is required to pass rigorous exams in the state in which he or she wishes to practice. I cannot overemphasize the barrier this presents to individual dentists. However, a dentist can overcome these barriers with enough time and effort and can choose a geographic location and still be able to practice his or her profession, even down to the size and makeup of the town or city desired. Unlike some careers, dentists are not transferred from location to location as is the norm in certain corporations. In other words, dentistry offers considerable flexibility in determining the type of practice and its locale.

What is the day of a typical general dentist like? Here is a two-day schedule you might find in any dentist's office:

	Monday		Tuesday
8:00a.m.	Jane Tree immediate denture	8:00a.m.	S. Lincoln examine tongue
8:15	Harry Young suture removal	8:15	Tony Wood seat sp maint
8:45	Ronnie Reague amalgams, N2O	8:45	Mrs. Redden Emergency
9:00	Debbie Wall 3 crowns	9:00	Donna Gates tongue swallow
10:15	Jim Crowely root canal #13, N2O	9:15	Joe White composites
10:45	Sally Joiner extraction #32	9:45	Philip Martell Check swelling
11:30	John Kally composites	10:00	Andy Paters perio surg.,N2O
12:00	Lunch with C.P.A.	11:00	Jane Tree check denture
1:00p.m.	William O'Keefe deliver partial	11:15	Ronnie Reague amalgams, N2O
1:15	Bill Green Post and core #19	11:45	Jennifer Addison

Time	Patient / Procedure	Time	Patient / Procedure
1:45	Jack Jones Change perio pack		consult with mother about frenectomy
2:00	Janice Jones root canal #8	12:00 1:00p.m.	Lunch David Absot reline denture
2:30	Myra Smith dry socket	1:15	Jerry Olson extract #1, 16,
2:45	Tommie Strait new patient, emerg		17, 32
3:00	Roger Jackson occlusal adjustment	2:15	Mrs. Moreland add tooth, partial
3:30	Owen Katzen deliver bridge	3:00	Richard Moreland crowns #7, 8, 9,
4:00	Mrs. Brown try-in denture	4:15	10 David Thomas
4:15	Pat Hotom recement crown #11	4:30	Check perio #3 Pat Hotom
4:30	Katie Meth amalgams		recement crown #11
		4:40	Mrs. Cody exam, lesion on
4:50	Larry Bue suture removal		lip
		4:45	Bob Jones. amalgam, N2O

This dentist was always busy, always meeting new challenges, with no time to be bored. Although constantly achieving and justifiably proud of his successful services, not once did the dentist feel glamorous in these two days. In fact, he or she may have felt a little unappreciated when the certified public accountant revealed the tax bill for the last quarter. Yet, for each patient, the dental experience was intensely personal, an unusual occurrence. The dentist was expected to perform the difficult techniques precisely and perfectly, each and every time. Each patient believed the dentist was aware of the latest developments in dental science as they applied to him or her. In addition, that pat on the shoulder or squeeze of the hand or little smile was needed to put the patient at ease. The elderly women and men appreciated the dentist's helping them out of the chair, although they could not have known that another patient was put on hold on the telephone for the few minutes this courtesy required. If the dentist cannot savor the humanness, the one-to-one contact, the "Thank-you, doctor," then this career will not bring joy.

The dentist is unlikely to have business training, but he or she will have to manage the complicated business of a practice. Even in clinic situations, the dentist is expected to oversee the auxiliary personnel. He or she has to know when to delegate authority, as much as is allowed within the law of the particular state of the practice. The future dentist may well realize that 99 percent of the personnel he or she will be around for many hours each day will be women. Not only is he or she ultimately responsible for these women's actions, but the dentist has certain obligations to the auxiliaries. Some states require that each employed person leaving the dental operation be given a copy of any radiation exposure she may have encountered. A former employee can hold the dentist responsible if that employee was not adequately and reasonably protected from hazards such as infectious diseases or mercury contamination.

Because of the lack of business expertise, the dentist is wise to employ specialists such as lawyers, certified public accountants, and insurance experts. Nevertheless, the dentist must acquaint him or herself with these areas, because any liability is his or hers. The dentist may not land in jail because of willful tax evasion, but he or she could end up owing thousands of dollars in taxes and penalties because of sloppy accounting. Some lawyers may not be as careful as they should be, and the dentist must be wise enough to think deeply before choosing a lawyer and acting on any legal advice given.

The dentist also has to set fees, payment policies, and collection policies. He or she will work with several insurance companies, and patients mistakenly expect dentists to be experts in the area of dental insurance. The dentist has to oversee the control of inventory, making sure fresh medications and medicaments are used. Of course, all the bills and payroll must be paid before the dentist can dare pay any salary to him or herself.

Like the general practitioner, the specialists also face these problems. The specialists hold either the DDS or DMD degree, but they have studied an additional two, three, or four years and have had to pass further board examinations. Of 137,817 practicing dentists, 27,563 have qualified as specialists in one of the eight dental specialties recognized by the American Dental Association:

Endodontics: commonly called "root canal therapy." An endodontist must complete additional hours in the study of the biology of the normal pulp and supporting structures, etiology, diagnosis, and prevention and treatment of diseases and injuries of the pulp and periradicular tissues.

Oral pathology: commonly known as "biopsy results." The oral pathologist studies the nature of diseases affecting the oral and adjacent structures. He or she uses clinical, microscopic, radiographic, biochemical, and other laboratory procedures to establish a diagnosis or gain other information to maintain the health of the patient.

Oral and maxillofacial surgery: commonly thought of as "jaw sugery" or "extractions." This specialist deals with the diagnosis and the surgical and adjunctive treatment of diseases, injuries, and defects of the oral and facial region.

Orthodontics: commonly known as "braces." An orthodontist is concerned with the supervision, guidance, and correction of the developing dentofacial structures. Orthodontics includes diagnosis, prevention, interception, and treatment of all forms of malocclusion of the teeth and their surrounding structures.

Periodontics: commonly called "gum treatment." A periodontist treats diseases and abnormalities and injuries of the tissues surrounding the teeth. These include the hard, boney tissue as well as the gums, mucosa and muscle attachments.

Prosthodontics: commonly called a "denture specialist." A prosthodontist restores and maintains the patient's oral functions, comfort, and appearances by the restoration of natural teeth or the replacement of missing teeth and contiguous tissues with artificial substitutes.

Dental public health: commonly called "disease control." This specialist prevents and controls dental diseases and promotes dental health through organized community efforts; he or she serves the community as a whole rather than the individual patient.

Some dentists prefer not to enter private practice nor to specialize. Many types of professional opportunities are available to a DDS or a DMD in administrative, educational, and research positions. For example, there are consulting positions with universities, insurance companies, and dental manufacturers. Many pharmaceutical and laboratory businesses employ dentists in research. He or she may work as a dentist or adviser in a government health agency or a private agency; some public schools and community agencies employ dentists on a full- or part-time basis. Many young dentists decide to enter the armed forces after dental school.

A distinct advantage to choosing dentistry as a career may be overlooked by young people: the advantages that come to the dentist's family. In the back of the student's mind is the idea that some day he or she will indeed have a spouse and children, but it is hard to imagine the over-

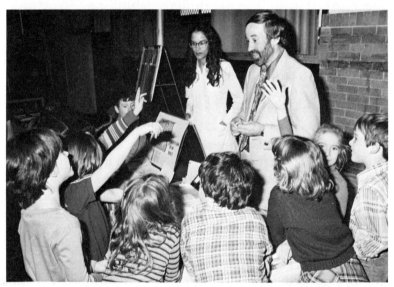

Dr. James B. Phillips and Dr. Jessica A. Rickert are the dental experts at a Health Fair at Pierce Elementary School. They volunteered to speak to over 350 students, that day, along with nine other health experts (William A. Strait Photography).

whelming influence their welfare will have on his or her life. Dentistry, more than any other branch of medicine, has the advantage of flexibility. A dentist can work part time or full time as the family needs dictate; when both the husband and the wife are working and the children are young, this option becomes more attractive. That is not to say that the patients' needs can be put off or taken lightly; however, the dentist can determine whether or not new patients will be added to the work load and even which procedures he or she will decide to refer. Very often, arrangements with a trusted colleague can be made so that the dentist will not have to be on call constantly. Thereby, adequate time for vacations and special events can be scheduled with the family in mind. A fully integrated life—professional and family—can only help to make a better dentist.

It almost goes without saying that the dentist's family will take great pride in his or her profession. The community looks to its dentists for leadership. There will be many requests for service, and any service rendered to society by the dentist always brings rewards for the family and spouse as well. As a dentist, the young man or woman can expect to know and influence other leaders in the community, in business, in other professions, and in the government. He or she must always remember to conduct him or herself with the utmost decorum, for he or she is always a representative of the profession. This representation—whether negative or positive—will also reflect on the dentist's family and spouse. On the other hand, the family and spouse must realize that the patient's needs will sometimes supersede their own needs or desires. When this happens, there should not be any resentment toward the patient or the dentist, because the dentist's choice is always clear. He or she will see to the needs of the patient. This is an infrequent occurrence in dentistry, but it is wise to have the spouse and family understand the dentist's responsibility before emergencies arise. The many opportunities dentistry opens to the spouse and family far outweigh the disadvantages.

An obvious concern when considering dentistry is the financial remuneration of the profession. Unless the young person knows a dentist quite well, he or she may not fully realize all the aspects involved. Dentists, especially young ones, are seldom rich. Certainly, they may be well off, and it is unlikely that they will want for the necessities of life, but it is also unlikely that dentistry will make anyone an easy millionaire. If wealth is a known desire for a student, he or she will have to consider other fields. Really, the best way to phrase it is as a "dentist's income earning *potential*"; the opportunity to earn a fine living is certainly there. The income of the average self-employed dentist in 1989 was $85,690, *1989 Survey of Dental Practice*, American Dental Association. But the dentist, especially the young dentist, is only earning when a patient is being treated. Even so, those dentists who work sixty or seventy hours a week trying to accumulate money will more likely become "rich" through investments rather than from direct payments from patients.

Most students don't realize the large expenditures the average young practitioner carries. Dental manufacturers give quotes from $75,000 to $250,000 as the start-up costs of a practice in 1990. Quite attractive to the young dentist is to purchase a retiring or moving dentist's practice, because the equipment, supplies, and patient load are already there. This is explored in greater detail in Chapter V, but basically these arrangements usually involve a price of 50 percent of the previous year's gross receipts minus debts. Final figures may be from $10,000 to $150,000, depending upon the practice. Some dentists continue to purchase retiring practices for six or seven years, incorporating those patients into their practice.

In Chapter IV we shall examine the graduating dental student's debt, but the average figure in 1990 was $45,550 for residents and $44,630 for non-residents. It is unlikely that anyone who is not independently wealthy would be able to borrow even more money to set up a practice. That is why many young dentists take paid employment or enter the armed services for two or three years after graduation. Another alternative is to work as an associate with the opportunity to "buy in" over a period of years.

It sounds as if dentistry can be an ideal career, doesn't it? For the right person, dentistry is indeed a great opportunity, an enjoyable art, and a rewarding service to humankind. However, there are certain frustrations in every job, and some are unique to dentistry. As I've tried to emphasize, the orientation of dentistry has to be in an intensely interpersonal, one-to-one direction. Certainly, this constant dealing with people can become quite wearying. A survey conducted by an Arizona consulting firm, Nexus Group, Inc.,[1] showed stress as the number one job-related complaint of dentists. One study, by Weinstein and associates in 1978, reported that dentists felt they had problems with 20 percent of their patients.[2] The most common complaint in that study was that a substantial number of patients did not appreciate the importance of optimal dental care. Another study in 1978 by Ingersoll and associates found the following to be specific problems encountered by dentists, in order of frequency: fee collections; fearful patients and a lack of cooperation in the dental chair; poor oral hygiene; ignorance of preventive care; failure to follow instructions; insurance paperwork; poorly behaved children; and broken, canceled, or late appointments.[3] In 1982 Corah and associates studied 376 dentists and found these frequent and bothersome problems: poor oral hygiene;

---

[1]Tsalikis, Penny, "Pain Control," *Dental Management,* June, 1982.

[2]Weinstein, P. W., and others, "Dentists' Perceptions of Their Patients: Relations to Quality of Care," *Journal of Public Health, Dentistry,* Vol. 38, pp. 10-21, 1978.

[3]Ingersoll, T. G., and others, "A Survey of Patients and Auxiliary Problems as they Relate to Behavioral Dentistry Curricula," *Journal of Dental Education,* Vol. 42, pp. 260-263, 1978.

broken, canceled, or late appointments; nonpayment for dental services; lack of cooperation in the dental chair; failure to care for dentures; failure to follow post-op instructions; failure to provide accurate history; and failure to wear dentures and biteplate.[4] Under the heading of uncooperative behavior in the chair were: showing unrealistic fear; not keeping mouth open; talking during procedures; jerking head away; excessive gagging; not appreciating dental treatment; questioning the dentist's judgment; criticizing the dentist; screaming; and grabbing the dentist's hand.

All dentists will agree that they have been frustrated by some items on this list at one time or another. Many of the behaviors show a lack of common courtesy and consideration and are simply inexcusable. But there are obnoxious people in the population at large with whom we all have to deal. A dentist must learn to put such actions into perspective and not to take them personally. It is unrealistic to expect people always to behave perfectly; in fact, a patient consumed by trauma, pain, infection, and anxiety may act completely out of character when he or she complains to the dentist. Can you ignore this less than ideal behavior? Can you tolerate people who may be out of control? Can you address and attack the tropisms called anxiety, fear, and cowardice rather than the people exhibiting them? Can you assess a situation, take charge, and rechannel the action? Do you tend to take negative reactions personally and dwell on disappointment, worrying, wondering, rehashing every detail?

Let me share with you a lesson I learned from a social worker whom I happened to observe in a different situation. He was a six-and-a-half-footer who found himself on the receiving end of a torrent of verbal abuse from a

---

[4]Corah, Norman L., Ph.D.; O'Shea, Robert L., Ph.D.; and Skeels, David, "Dentists' Perceptions of Problem Behaviors in Patients," *Journal of the American Dental Association*, Vol. 104, No. 6, pp. 829–883, June, 1982.

disheveled, overwrought woman. She called him every name in the book, ending with,

"You're the ugliest so-and-so I ever laid eyes on!"

His reply? "You're right, Ms. X. I'm so ugly that I broke my bathroom mirror this morning. I'm trying to save up enough money so that I can see a plastic surgeon right away."

He was able to disarm her wrath without raising a finger—or even his voice. He always spoke calmly and slowly and politely as he addressed Ms. X. She could not rile him, and so she stopped trying.

Although few dentists will have to deal with as irksome a situation as this, it is unrealistic to expect that a dentist will never encounter an irate or irrational patient. A young person would be wise to anticipate how he or she will react to unpleasant situations. More important, he or she ought to put these infrequent occurrences in perspective and to realize that the majority of patients are just like you and me—enjoyable, interesting, and unique persons.

For certain persons dentistry simply would be the wrong career choice, an expensive, agonizing mistake. After completing four years of undergraduate work and four years of dental school, after passing the rigorous board examinations and procuring a place as an associate, why did one young man leave the profession after three frustrating clinical years?

We shall call him "Dr. XYZ." Here is our interview:

Dr. Rickert: When did you graduate from dental school?

Dr. XYZ: In 1970. That was about the best time there was for starting a dental practice.

Dr. Rickert: What had made you decide to pursue dentistry?

Dr. XYZ: My grandfather was a dentist, and my mother was a dental hygienist for some time before she had children. I knew I wanted to be a professional, and I am good at the sciences. I enjoy work that requires manual dexterity.

Dr. Rickert: How did you like dental school?

Dr. XYZ: Actually, it was pretty much as I had expected it to be, although harder. Yet I realized that the school was trying to train us in an extremely difficult field and that the courses had to be hard to prepare us for dentistry.

Dr. Rickert: Do you feel that dental school did in fact prepare you?

Dr. XYZ: Oh yes, definitely, for the dental diagnosis and treatment required for the general population. For the techniques, yes.

Dr. Rickert: How did you like dentistry?

Dr. XYZ: I did like it. There were some things about practice for which I was not prepared, such as dealing with the paperwork, insurance companies. Business aspects.

Dr. Rickert: But you did like the dentistry itself?

Dr. XYZ: Generally, yes. I did feel frustrated at times that the patients did not appreciate the fine dental restorations I was providing for them. I found it stressful to have to do a one-half job on patients who were extremely fearful. These are frustrations all dentists learn to deal with.

Dr. Rickert: What was the single most important reason you left dentistry?

Dr. XYZ: There were two major reasons. First was AIDS. I have always been concerned about hepatitis and herpes, and I maintained the most sterile and clean environment possible.

Dr. Rickert: But the Centers for Disease Control informs us that if we use barrier techniques such as eye goggles, masks, and rubber gloves it is virtually impossible to contract AIDS. That and careful sterilization techniques should protect us.

Dr. XYZ: Yes, yes. I used gloves and eye protection and masks. I know that AIDS is transmitted sexually and not by casual contact. But face it, dentistry is NOT casual contact; it is intimate contact. And AIDS is transmitted by blood. In dentistry we deal with blood all day as well as saliva.

Dr. Rickert: What about the type of population pool your patients came from?

Dr. XYZ: I don't believe there are IV drug users in my community. There *are* many gays. I never paid much attention to them; you know: live and let live. But I decided that I would try to keep gays out of my practice, if at all possible, when AIDS surfaced. Then the government stepped in and classified AIDS patients as "handicapped," saying that health professionals cannot discriminate to keep them out of our practices. And the AIDS patients will not identify themselves so that we can take special precautions such as double gloving.

Dr. Rickert: But medical science has shown us that with care it is not necessary to discriminate against AIDS patients, that they can be safely treated in our offices. Also, discrimination against them is the major cause of their not identifying themselves.

Dr. XYZ: That is correct. But remember, this was back in 1981, 1982, when nothing was known about the disease except that it was deadly.

But who can guarantee that every glove I put on is 100 percent free of microscopic holes? What if I have chapped hands the one day I get a glove with a hole in it? I myself may forget just one time and touch my eye with a finger that is not sterile? Will my assistant disinfect the instrument counter in the lab each and every time? What about the commercial dental labs I send my cases to: will they use every sterilization technique available? All it takes is one small error.

Don't get me wrong. I'm not against gays or hemophiliacs or even AIDS patients. I am very sorry that this disease has become manifest. I am very sorry for the people who have the disease. I wish there was a cure; I certainly don't want anybody to suffer. I don't think gays "deserve" this disease, or any disease. I just personally do not wish to put myself at risk for catching this disease or for bringing it home to my family.

Dr. Rickert: Yes, we are all nervous about AIDS. But you mentioned another reason for leaving dentistry.

Dr. XYZ: Yes, the malpractice crisis. So many doctors and dentists are being sued for complications or failure of treatment. Even a frivolous lawsuit is devastating for the doctor.

Dr. Rickert: Have you been sued?

Dr. XYZ: Oh no, but I have had patients threaten me, especially when I've had to go after payment. I have been able to talk to these disgruntled people and convince them that there is no basis for their threats. If I were to be sued, I am convinced the suit would have nothing to do with the dentistry involved, but rather would reflect the litigious society we live in. People think the way to settle differences is through the courts.

Dr. Rickert: What about the costs of liability insurance?

Dr. XYZ: Whew! I don't have to tell you that the rates are sky high. In the last three years my rate went up 500 percent! I have never been sued, but since I first began practicing my liability insurance rate has risen 1800 percent! I realize that inflation has to be taken into consideration, but even at these astronomical costs some dentists and specialists cannot even get liability coverage.

Dr. Rickert: But the huge increase is usually passed on to the patients. I guess if society wants to be litigious it will have to pay for it.

Dr. XYZ: That's right. Dental and medical fees are sky high and will continue to escalate as long as the liability crisis continues. But another concern I had was the eroding of the doctor/patient relationship. With so many lawsuits reported in the media, patients have become antagonistic toward doctors. I think some patients even try to trip up a doctor, try to get rich off a lawsuit.

In fact, I had reached a point where with each new patient I was asking myself: "Is this the one who's going to get me?" New patients were probably asking themselves the same thing about me.

I hate the fact that there is such an adversarial relationship between doctor and patient. I want to help people and to have people trust me. I want to trust my patients so that we can work together to improve their dental health. I honestly feel that the joy is gone from practice.

Dr. Rickert: Now that you've decided to leave dentistry, what will you do?

Dr. XYZ: Luckily, some things I've invested in are paying off. My sister and I opened a fast-food franchise six years ago. We've opened several other similiar franchises, and our executive officer is leaving, so I'm going to run all four stores. We're going to open three new stores in the next three years, so I'll be busy.

Dr. Rickert: And your practice?

Dr. XYZ: I was able to find a young dentist to purchase my practice. I am financing him through a land contract. He's eager to have a go at dentistry, and I know he'll do well.

Dr. Rickert: Thank you for your time, and I hope you do well in your future endeavors.

III

For years I suffered with headaches. They weren't often severe, but there was always the constant heaviness, the threat of exploding pain at any time. I had been tested for high blood pressure, low blood sugar, poor eyesight, spinal curvature, and so on, and finally was sent to a neurologist, who looked for tumors and such. A psychiatrist told me I was too tense and to loosen up and take some Valium. It helped somewhat.

I hadn't been to the dentist for a while because of my headache problem, but a molar cracked, so I knew I had to get in to see him. He updated my health questionnaire, because it had been three years since my last visit. That's when I mentioned the headaches and the treatment I was under. He began asking me questions, like when were the headaches the worst, what time of day; where did the pain start, which side. Did the pain move? Then he asked if my teeth ever ached in the morning. Yes, quite often, especially in the morning, but it was never severe, and it disappeared by the time I had eaten breakfast. Dr. Traverse asked if he could examine my "bite." It was pretty hard for him to do because my jaw muscles were like bands of steel, they were so tight. When he asked me to open and close really big, I felt some pain when he pressed gently on my jaw joint. He suggested that much of my headache problem could be coming from a bad bite.

I was willing to try just about anything, so I let him make

a soft, plastic bite plane. Dr. Traverse wanted me to wear it all the time, but I decided not to wear it to work because it interfered with my speech and was very cumbersome. My mouth produced a lot of extra saliva, trying to adapt to the big thing. (It didn't look that big when I held it in the palm of my hand.) He informed me that this was a temporary appliance, just to allow my jaw muscles to rest and relax so that he could evaluate my bite better. In about ten days, my headaches were diminishing. Then the doctor began to adjust my bite by spot grinding on my back teeth. I was pretty nervous about it at first, but it was not uncomfortable, and the little bit he ground off was not noticeable, especially since he always made sure to smooth and polish the teeth afterwards. There were four or five such appointments. In that time, about two months, I had only three headaches, and they were not severe. Dr. Traverse then made me a hard bite plane to be worn at night. It was smaller, but in some ways I liked the soft bite plane better.

The dentist also explained to me how stress and tension are transmitted through the brain to the teeth, causing certain people to grind or clench their teeth in an attempt to wear down the high spots. He advised me to begin exercising regularly, and even gave me some relaxation techniques to use whenever I feel stressful. I am not totally "cured" because I still get an occasional headache. But I sure do feel a lot better about myself, and I haven't taken a Valium in four months now.

Ms. Linda Thelin is a thirty-year-old secretary, a divorcee with three children. Although it was hard for her to find time to follow all of Dr. Traverse's advice, she made the effort to do so. He wanted her also to give up her eight cups of coffee and pack of cigarettes per day, but she has not been willing to do so. Since her headaches are virtually gone, she will continue with the hard bite plane and regular checkups to "check her bite."

Chapter III

Qualifications of a Young Person

Since dentistry is a science, the student must have a high degree of proficiency in all the science subjects. Math, as a basis for the other studies, has to be a stronghold. Physics, chemistry, and biology should have a cumulative 3.0 grade point average in high school before the student can even hope to master the undergraduate courses requisite to applying to dental school. A thorough command of English and an excellent reading ability cannot be overemphasized. In dental school the student will be required to master all his or her textbooks, lecture handouts, and notes, as well as volumes of articles in the dental literature. He or he will also be expected to hand in papers of professional quality on a regular basis. Any graduate study, as an example, for the specialties, requires further thesis papers and special reports; it is assumed that all of these papers will be neatly typed.

In addition, some admissions committees are seeking students who have a strong background in the humanities, such as the social sciences and the arts. The high school student must be encouraged to work to his potential in all subjects; likewise, the college student is wise to excel and to study hard. The I.Q. of the student is not given much weight when he or she applies to dental school; the past performance is.

In 1989 there were 4,964 applicants for 3,979 places in American dental schools.

Even some qualified students were rejected.

Another measure of the student's ability is the Dental Aptitude Test, which is covered in depth in Chapter IV. Suffice it to say that the students with higher scores will have a greater chance of being accepted to a dental school.

An important talent is manual dexterity. The vast majority of dentists spend considerable time manipulating fine and precious objects. A dentist's hands are also diagnostic instruments; subtle differences in tissues are sensed through the fingers. More than many other healing arts, dentistry requires the laying on of hands in order for the patient to be made whole again. When a patient comes to you in distress, you will possess the ability in your mind and hands to set things right for that patient. It's an awesome privilege. For those without the manual talents, it will also become a huge frustration. If you already know that your hands are not capable of delicate technique, it is best to consider another career. Those who discover this frustration after graduation from dental school should consider work in dental administration or consultation.

Some anthropologists state that mankind's advancement to superiority in the animal kingdom came about because of our highly developed brains and hands. Dentistry challenges the student to excel in both areas.

Although intellectual and manual ability are essential before one considers dentistry as a career, a student's personality will largely determine his or her success. A doctor must possess a genuine love for all humanity. He or she must be calm, patient, compassionate, and slow to anger. A stable, well-developed personality is the basis for the tremendous psychic energy necessary to face day to day physical contact with many people. Inherently, a dentist has to be meticulous and able to concentrate on the tiniest, precise details for long periods of time. A dentist has to possess the tenacity to stick to any job until it is completed satisfactorily. There are not many instantaneous rewards in dentistry.

Are you a person who basks in others' approval? Do you need constant attention? Does your ego need massaging? Dentistry does not often offer these compensations. Very few communities would doubt the importance of their dentist, but don't expect any parades in the dentist's honor. The public is not waiting with open arms and fanfare for the recent dental graduate; you, the expert, can become accustomed to being taken for granted. The dentist must be satisfied *within him or herself.*

We are busy talking about becoming a "successful dentist," but let's take a moment to consider the idea of "success." What is your definition of success? Each person must define this for him or herself. Do not choose dentistry or any other career because you identify with the life-style it offers. A man or woman must realize that the work itself is the essential ingredient for day-to-day satisfaction throughout one's life. We must have a goal before we can realize it. Success implies the concepts of "prospering, flourishing, and thriving." How do these adjectives apply to your goal?

Carefully think over the following questions:

Do you enjoy *recognition* as a member of a larger organization? You've been a member of a larger organization for most of your life, your school. You know that it offers you some instant identification as well as protection. The other students' reputations, achievements, and failures reflect on you as soon as you say what school you attend. As a private practitioner, you are not afforded this mantle. When patients question your office policy or your treatment, you must be able to say "*I* do not allow that," or "*I* have decided to do so and so." Then you'll have to stand alone as you explain your decision. For this very reason, some dental students decide to stay on as researchers or teachers at their dental schools, for they can then call on the greater authority of the school.

Do you enjoy close *friendship* with those with whom you work? As the authority figure in the private office, it is very unlikely that you'll form deep friendships with the personnel. Simply put, it can be "lonely at the top." Remember, most auxiliary personnel will be female, and male dentists who form close relationships with these women may well run into conflicts. Female dentists, also, must remember that it is far harder to fire one's "best friend" than it is to fire "the receptionist." For this reason, many dentists prefer to work in hospital settings or group practices, where there are many colleagues with whom to form warm friendships.

Are you a *competitive* person? As a dentist, you may well be the final authority figure, but at the same time it is essential to be able to work cooperatively with your personnel, with other medical and dental doctors, and, of course, with the patients. The competitive spirit that embodies the idea of winning by beating or defeating an opponent does not have a place in the dental setting.

What do the terms *power, authority, and influence* mean to you? Can you accept the responsibility that goes with those concepts? Can you not abuse the position you may some day hold as a dentist? In fact, some people are quite uncomfortable holding positions of authority over anyone; these people abdicate their authority subconsciously, rationalizing that "everything will work out by itself." Things rarely work out by themselves, but rather require conscious decision-making. Can you do this and still be able to admit to errors in your judgment? Can you possess power and not let it possess you? Can you delegate authority, as much as is allowed by the dental law in your state? In medicine especially, doctors are often accused of having a "god complex." Do you think you can help your fellow human beings better with or without having a "god complex"?

Do you seek *excitement*? Adventure? Dentistry is not exciting, really, although the rewards can be great. It may even be downright discouraging at times. Don't expect a TV series to be aired or a Broadway show to be produced about the adventures of dentistry. Dentistry is always changing, but the challenge comes from the human, scientific, and aesthetic variables that come into play with each patient. Comparing dentistry to sky-diving is just not possible.

What about *physical challenge*? Physical prowess? Dentistry is performed sitting down, in a small space. Difficult physical procedures require some muscular strength, but they especially require muscular control. As a woman dentist, fellows often comment to me, "But you don't look strong enough to pull a tooth." If brute force were all that were needed to extract a tooth, I'd just put a speedy end to that conversation. Although it seems as if it would be easy to become overweight and physically "soft," most dentists find that physical activity plays an important part in their life-style; the dental societies themselves sponsor such activities as golf leagues, tennis camps, and jogging classes. Certainly, most dentists can afford the options of after-hours sports. In addition, certain muscle masses have to be strengthened, such as the arms, the wrist and finger muscles, the neck muscles, and the back. Dentists a few decades ago suffered from curved spines and varicose veins and fallen arches, but modern techniques make it possible to practice dentistry quite comfortably for long periods of time with little or no direct physical harm to the dentist.

How important is *time freedom* to you? Although a dentist is often on call and has to make sure his or her patients will be cared for, nevertheless most dentists in private practice can and do set their own business hours. Nighthawks may choose to work from 1:00 p.m. until 9:00 p.m., and early birds can work from 7:00 a.m. until 3:00 p.m. Don't worry, the patients may even prefer these odd hours. Dentists can and do take from two to eight weeks of vacation time per year. It would be unusual to find a dentist who takes off eight weeks in a row, but it's not unusual for one to take off two weeks every three or four months. As long as the dentist remembers that the patient's needs have to be met, he or she is afforded much more time freedom than professionals or executives employed by large companies or firms. However, some people cannot function comfortably without a stringent time schedule imposed upon them by others. In other words, with too much time freedom, they never seem to accomplish anything. Into which category do you fit?

How important is *geographic freedom* to you? Dentists can work wherever there are people. It's not quite as simple as that, for there are varying licensing requirements from state to state. However, a dentist who knows where he or she wishes to reside can make it happen. Or he or she can reverse that decision and move again.

How important is your *moral obligation* to you? For religious persons this is an especially important question. Many occupations cannot be easily reconciled to the edification of deep moral convictions. Dentistry, while not a spiritual endeavor per se, does lend itself to an interweaving with one's moral goals. Old and young dentists alike may choose to take off a year or two to serve as missionary dentists, in church-related clinics, or in the Peace Corps. The feeling of meeting a real need through dentistry can take on special significance for these people.

Besides the scholastic, manual, and personality requirements, the sudent is expected to have other talents and interests. Music, art, theater, and sport experiences are important; special awards and achievements in these areas demonstrate that the young person is a well-rounded individual.

For the high school and college student, work history can be beneficial, especially if it has shown that the student has a certain empathy for the patients he or she will encounter in the health field. If the student can find employment in a dental or medical setting, this will be the best basis for his or her career decision. The work record will also be scrutinized when applying to dental school. Did the student change jobs constantly, after only two or three weeks? Was the employee late or absent a lot? What raises were given? Don't be surprised if no one on the admissions committee of a dental school cares whether or not you liked your boss. You will be judged by your performance.

A young person can pursue activities with the conscious intent of preparing for a career in dentistry. The Red Cross and other health-related agencies take volunteers as young as fourteen. This experience will let you know if you can like sick people. How will you react to suffering? Emotionally, can you overlook the sights, sounds, and smells of illness? Other volunteer activity in the varied health fields can help you make up your mind which direction you ought to take.

Since a dentist encounters all age groups, a young man or woman should consider interacting with preschoolers for many hours. Does their crying bother you? Can you help the child overcome his or her fears? Oldsters will also be encountered; most are sage conversationalists, but there are some senior citizens whose favorite pastime is complaining about aches and pains and a hard life. Does that bother you? Can you steer their energy in other directions? Can you identify with oldsters' diminished physical capacity? Physically handicapped people need dental care; will you be willing to install special access ramps so that they can easily be wheeled in? Do the uncontrolled movements and spasms of some handicaps bother you? What about the physical characteristics of various deformities? Can you sit close to and touch these special patients for long periods of time? What about people with emotional or mental handicaps? A thirty-year-old man with the mental capacity of a five-year-old can be shocking the first time you see him. So can an autistic three-year-old who simply rocks back and forth, back and forth, back and forth. How will you deal with this child's dental needs? Volunteering to work with some of these people will help prepare the young person for his or her role as a doctor.

As for manual dexterity, any endeavor in which the hands are used can only help to ingrain the neuromuscular tracks in the student's cerebral cortex, making future training that much easier. Sculpting small figures is helpful, as is sewing. Soldering an intricate electronic circuit board can improve the delicacy of one's touch. Model building and woodworking can improve eye-hand coordination. Painting heightens aesthetic awareness, as does jewelry design. Pottery and ceramics enable the young person to strengthen the hands as well as to foster creativity. Even car mechanics develop eye-hand coordination and the muscles in the hands. Some students purchase special exercise equipment to strengthen the hand muscles, but most of the activities mentioned will develop the hands enough if they are pursued actively.

The visual ability of the dentist is important. First and foremost, do not compromise your vision by reading or working in poor light or by holding books too close. Follow any advice the eye doctor gives you.

The dentist must be able to visualize intricate aesthetic procedures upside down and backwards. A course in drafting and mechanical drawing can help the student to develop his or her visualization talents, as can perspective, map, and architectural drawing. Blueprinting is another skill that can tax the young person. The visualization portions of the Dental Aptitude Test is described in a later chapter, but many students find it the most difficult part of the test simply because they have never challenged this skill before. Even those with natural visualization talents can improve with practice. Jigsaw puzzles develop this skill, as do games of eye-hand coordination. Some prospective students begin by performing this seemingly simple exercise: obtain any line drawing, even from an old coloring book, and place it on a table in front of you. Now put a mirror in front of you and the paper, with the reflecting surface toward you so that you can see the paper in the mirror. Attempt to trace the line drawing by looking in the mirror only. Do not look directly at the paper. It may take quite a while before you can trace a picture perfectly. Then it's time to move on to a more difficult picture. Next try writing your name. You might even try to build something while looking in the mirror.

One of the best ways to appreciate the daily life of a dentist is to visit one's office for a few hours. You might begin by approaching your own dentist or a friend of the family who happens to be a dentist. If you cannot do that, call your local dental society and explain that you're interested in a dental career and would like to talk to a practicing dentist. Write a short note to him or her, asking for an appointment. Of course, you must be willing to go when it's convenient for the dentist; this will most likely be after 5:00 p.m. Arrive on time, dressed nicely. Ask permission to ask some questions about dentistry:

1. What dental school did the dentist attend? What was it like?
2. Does the dentist like being a dentist? Would he or she go into dentistry if it were to be done over again?

3. Would the dentist advise his or her children to go into the field?
4. What was his or her day like, today?
5. What are his or her goals for the future?
6. Ask if he or she has dentist friends who would be willing to talk to you.
7. Ask if it would be possible for you to observe the office operation for two or three hours, at his or her convenience. State that you have your own white coat to wear to the office. Ask if you can bring a notebook with you.
8. Thank the dentist for the time and information.

On the appointed day, be sure to arrive a few minutes early so that if the dentist has had to make some adjustments in the schedule of patients for the day, your visit will easily fit in. Dress neatly, as if you were going to church, not to a party or dance. Make sure that your hair is out of the way; even clean hair houses bacteria, and it should not be necessary for the dentist to point this out. Put on your white coat when you are in the office proper. The dentist will probably ask the dental assistant to show you around and to place you where you'll be inconspicuous. Do not pester the dentist or try to impress him or her with your I.Q. The dental personnel are not interested in your situation, but are concentrating on the patient procedures at hand. Quietly stay where you have been placed; in the notebook you have brought with you write down any questions you might have, for later. If the dentist wants to point out certain things to you, consider yourself fortunate; do not expect this privilege. Do not fidget or sigh; keep a poker face and do not grimace or frown. If a particular phase of treatment makes you feel uneasy, avert your eyes to a distant corner of the office or count the ceiling tiles. Do not faint!

When it is time to leave, quietly thank the doctor. As soon as you get home, be sure to write a thank-you note to the entire staff and doctor. I mention this obvious courtesy, because the student needs to know that it is in fact inconvenient for the doctor to allow him or her in the office. Also, other young people may make the same request of the dentist, and the student's inappropriate actions could very well jeopardize someone else's chances of visiting the office in the future.

Another way to familiarize yourself with the dental field is to visit a dental school. Most schools set aside a careers day on a weekend and make special effort to tailor a program to the young adult's questions; usually, dental students act as guides for small groups. Even if you cannot make it on the careers day, do visit the school; dental schools expect this and are set up to answer questions about dentistry. If your parents would like to attend, by all means have them do so. However, this is *your* endeavor, so do not ask your mother or father to make arrangements for your visit. You call the school, you set up the date and appointment; you handle the arrival and introductions; you thank the dental students or professors who give you their time. Be sure to ask any questions you have; do not be afraid that a question might be "stupid." You cannot have too much information when trying to decide whether or not a particular career is correct for you. Besides, even if a question actually is stupid, you only need to ask it once, and then you'll know. Ask the dental students questions about the nonstudent aspects of their lives as well.

1. What is the housing in the area like? Does the school provide adequate housing?
2. Are most of the students commuters? Is the public or university transportation adequate?
3. Are support facilities such as day-care centers available?
4. What about cost of living—is it high or low compared to your hometown?

5. What about the environment itself? It is as hard for a big-city youngster to be stranded out in the boondocks as it is for a small-town student to find him or herself in the midst of a teeming metropolitan city.

6. Some schools attempt to offer recreational facilities for the students and faculty; others make no such facilities available.

7. Ask about affiliations with other medical complexes such as hospitals, nursing homes, clinics, and prisons.

If the dental student has the time and seems willing, you might ask even more questions about his experiences at the school:

1. Is he or she happy with the choice of dentistry as a career?

2. Is the school adequately preparing the student for a career in dentistry?

3. What is the best thing about dental school for that student?

4. What is the worst thing about dental school for that student?

5. What has been the hardest thing in dental school for that student? What class is the hardest for dental students as a whole?

6. What has been the easiest thing about dental school for that student? What class is the easiest for dental students as a whole?

7. What advice would the dental student give a younger person to improve the chances of entering dental school.

It's not surprising that most dental students are more than willing to talk about themselves and their dental school if the inquiring young person demonstrates a respectful inquisitiveness.

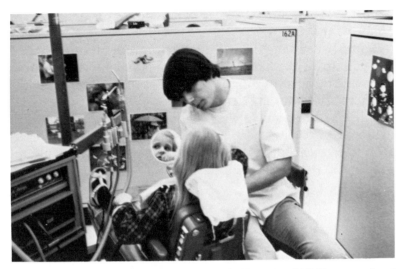

Dental students in the junior and senior years at the University of Michigan are assigned individual cubicles in which to provide dental services. (University of Michigan School of Dentistry, Photographic Department).

To familiarize yourself further with the dental field, you might consider visiting a dental lab in your area. A short tour of the facility is all that is necessary. If the laboratory technician has the time, you might ask him or her what it is like to work with dentists. Another question might be why did the laboratory technician choose this field rather than becoming a dentist? As a matter of fact, many young people have become dentists after working a summer or two in a commercial dental laboratory. You might ask the owner if he hires students on a part-time basis, but do not attempt to turn this short tour into a job prospect, or the owner might doubt your honest intentions.

Another source of information is the local dental supply house. These commercial enterprises are the "supermarkets" of the dentists. In addition to supplying sundries, however, these businesses also supply expertise in setting up dental offices and clinics. You might ask for prices of certain types of standard dental equipment, and how a new dentist finances this. Ask in what direction dentistry is going in the future.

You can see that there are many sources of information for you to tap. Share all the input available with those adults who are important in your life, such as your parents, teachers, and church friends. They may have insight as to whether or not your talents would be suited for the health field and for dentistry in particular. But be reminded that no one else can integrate all the information available to you and that no one else can make any career decision for you.

IV

When I was nine years old I was in a car accident, and my mouth hit the dashboard. Both of my front teeth were knocked out. The doctor at the hospital found out I was not otherwise injured and called for a dentist to come and examine me. The dentist asked if I had the teeth with me, but no one had thought to pick them up. So he sewed up my gums and sent me home with a prescription for an antibiotic.

At first I was the center of attention because I had lost my teeth. Then nobody noticed it for a couple of years, because all the kids were losing or just getting their teeth. By the time I was about ten, it was obvious to everyone that I had a problem. But I was pretty good at basketball, so the kids didn't hassle me too much.

In my senior year at high school, the missing teeth really bothered me a lot. I knew the girls liked me, but I just could not bring myself to ask them out for dates. I did not smile for my senior picture that fall, but presented a stone face.

Finally I got up enough nerve to go see a dentist. My family was not likely to see the dentist if there were no problems. Anyway, this Dr. Clement was a very nice, kind old man with a little white hair left. He examined my teeth and was surprised that I had only two little cavities in the molars, since I had not seen a dentist for at least eight years. I told him that what I really wanted to talk about was the missing front teeth. He explained about partial

47

dentures and bridgework, and their relation to the maturing of teeth. At that time, my teeth were still pretty immature, according to him. I told him I wanted the bridge. Then he told me the price. It was much more than I expected, but I could understand why once he explained the delicate treatments and all the time involved and the use of gold to build the whole thing. Still, it was all I could do to fight back the tears, I wanted that bridge so much.

Dr. Clement must have sensed what was going through my mind because he said, "Son, let's see if we can't work something out by the time you graduate from high school."

I did have an after-school job, and I was working more that summer, so he and I worked out a payment schedule over the next six months. He began the treatment as soon as I had paid him $100. I realize now that that would not even have begun to cover his costs if I defaulted and didn't finish paying him. I don't exactly know why he took a chance on me, being that he was a white doctor and I was a black kid.

I tell you, once he cemented that bridge, I was a changed person! I couldn't wait for college that fall. I was going on a basketball scholarship, and the dentist advised me always to wear a mouthguard to protect the bridge. Since I had paid for it, I was sure going to protect it.

I had to take extra jobs that summer, lawn-cutting, hauling, and even baby-sitting, because I wanted to prove to Dr. Clement that I could keep my promise and pay it off by the time I left for college. That was the best investment I ever made.

Derrick Daniels graduated from college and went on to get a master's degree in business. He realized that he didn't have a secure future in professional basketball. The bridge Dr. Clement placed for him is still sound, and Derrick's adjacent teeth have not darkened yet as the dentist had advised him they eventually will as Derrick gets older. At that time, he may have to have the bridge replaced.

Chapter IV

Educational Requirements and Financial Considerations

The educational requirements for entering the dental profession are similar to those for entering any health field. The precollege curriculum in high school should be followed. If, however, you are an older student who did not complete the precollege course in high school and you have now decided to enter a health field, you can enroll in junior college classes to strengthen your background. Be sure to consult a predental counselor who can guide you in the appropriate courses to pursue. Most dental schools will not accept more than two years of junior college experience; and you'll have to attend one or more years at an accredited college. regardless of how excellent your junior college grade point is.

For the student now in high school, the following can serve as a guide to adequate preparation for college and dental school:

1. Four years of college-prep English, including grammar, American and English literature, and a writing course.
2. Four years of college-prep mathematics courses, including algebra, plane and solid geometry, and, if possible, calculus.
3. Four years of science to include biology, botany, chemistry, and physics.

4. Two or three years of a foreign language.
5. Two or three years of history, including world history and American history as well as the required American government classes.
6. A year or two of social sciences.
7. Other classes such as computers, mechanical drawing, drafting, or architectural drawing. These talents are being used more and more in the dental field.
8. As many classes in the arts as you can fit around the heavy schedule already outlined. Pursue these other endeavors even if you have to do so on your own time and without credit. They include music, art, theater, and sports. In the previous chapter, there are suggestions as to other volunteer or work experience that will help you prepare for a health career. If these activities interfere with the required school work, it is best to drop them until summer.

The high school student who is serious about entering the health field should strive to maintain a B or a 3.0 grade point average. This will prepare him or her to compete with other students who are vying for a place in the professional schools; but, more important, the hard work necessary in pursuing these subjects and maintaining a 3.0 average will prepare the young person for the hard work and constant concentration required in the dental field. If the student feels that he or she cannot maintain this intensity throughout his or her life, dentistry is not the right field to consider entering.

In college or junior college, a 3.0 or B average must be maintained, although some dental schools set the grade point average requirement at 2.7. The predental requirements vary from two to three to four years of undergraduate study; the best way to find out the school requirements is to write to the specific school or to the American Dental Association for information. A predental counselor will advise you to take the following in the years of college as preparation for most dental schools' requirements:

1. English. One full year or the equivalent of six semester hours or nine quarter hours.
2. Chemistry. Two full years or the equivalent of sixteen hours or twenty-four quarter hours. This has to include one year of inorganic chemistry and one full year of organic chemistry including the full laboratory work that accompanies those courses.
3. Biological science. One full year or the equivalent of eight hours or twelve quarter hours. At least four of these hours should include an advanced course in zoology, and the full laboratory work accompanying the courses. Botany is not recommended as part of the science requirement.
4. Physics. A full year or eight semester hours or twelve quarter hours, with the accompanying laboratory work.
5. Mathematics. One full year or eight semester hours or twelve quarter hours.
6. The remainder of the undergraduate years may be filled with courses in the social sciences, fine arts, and humanities. Psychology is strongly suggested. Courses in "nonscientific" subjects such as music, education, religion, drawing, design, and journalism are allowed to a maximum of eight credit hours or twelve quarter hours. In addition, since running a dental practice is very much like running a business, the young person would be wise to pick up a few classes in practice/business administration, because no such courses are given in the dental schools.

Although it would be wise to check with the dental school you are interested in as to its actual undergraduate requirements, you ought to realize that in 1989, 62 percent of students entering all dental schools in the United States had a baccalaureate degree, 19 percent had completed three years of undergraduate training, and 10 percent had no more than two years of predental education. The remainder of entering students, 9 percent, had completed further education, with either a master's or a PhD degree.

Nineteen American dental schools officially require two years of undergraduate work, forty schools require three years, and two require four years.[1][2]

The prospective student must realize that there is virtually no cross-over between the various dental disciplines. In other words, courses in dental hygiene, dental assisting, and dental technology are not considered suitable to fulfill any part of the minimum academic total required for admission to a school of dentistry. Therefore, a young person, probably a woman, who has made a wrong career decision at the level of graduation from high school and finds that dentistry itself rather than an auxiliary function is more suitable for her, will discover that she has extensive backtracking to do in course work, time, and money. In effect, this rigid separation of study locks the young person, probably a woman, into a mold that will allow her considerably less autonomy, financial reward, and power throughout her life. There have been many auxiliary personnel who, at the age of thirty, for example, realized that they had the potential all along to become a fine dentist but never considered the profession. Although it has been done, it is unlikely that the goal of becoming a dentist will ever be reached, since most women at that age find themselves with other overriding responsibilities such as marriage and young children. Returning to the stage of an entering freshman in college, financially, emotionally, and time-wise, may become a moot point. How much better it would be if all young people, male and female, could choose the course of study that will challenge and reward them the most throughout their lives

---

[1] University of Michigan School of Dentistry, *Bulletin, 1982–1984*, Vol. 11, No. 22.
[2] University of Michigan School of Dentistry, "Dentistry."

without stereotypically being molded into a career because of narrow-minded expectations based on sex.

The cost of a dental education is high. Serious thought must be given as to how one can finance it. Three state schools do not charge tuition to state residents; other states charge residents less than nonresidents. The lowest tuition charged to residents is $1906, and the highest tuition charged to nonresidents is $27,894 per year. The average first-year tuition and general fee costs in the 1989/1990 school year was between $9,281 and $13,954.[3] Added to this are living expenses, books, and supplies.

In the first year a dental student can expect to pay between $3,000 and $4,000 for instruments and materials, between $500 and $700 for books and supplies, and between $100 and $200 for uniforms and university fees. In the second year of study, the student will pay between $1,800 and $2,500 for instruments and materials, between $400 and $600 for books and supplies, and between $100 and $200 for uniforms and university fees. In the third year, he or she can expect to pay between $1,000 and $1,400 for instruments and materials, between $400 and $450 for books and supplies, and between $100 and $200 for uniforms and fees. In the fourth year, the student pays between $300 and $500 for books and supplies, between $100 and $200 for uniforms and university fees, and between $100 and $200 for instruments and materials.[4]

The dental student should not expect to work during the academic school year, so he or she will have to obtain the necessary funds from summer employment, parents, and savings. Scholarships as well as loans are available, and the serious sudent must write to the dental school he or she is considering or to the American Dental Association for information on financial aid. However, the vast majority of

---

[3] American Dental Association. Annual Report: Dental Education, 1989/1990.
[4] American Dental Association *Journal*, "Dental Education, 1981–1982," Vol. 104, pp. 882–887, June, 1982.

graduating dentists leave dental school with a substantial debt from their four years of study. The average indebtedness of 1989 dental school graduates was $45,550, according to a survey by the A.D.A. Select Committee. In fact, 26.7 percent had a debt of more than $50,000. This indebtedness becomes a major factor in the type of work sought upon graduation; since various types of employment in government may erase some or all of a student's debt in addition to the wages paid, many students serve the government for two to five years.

Although there are many explanations as to why it might be so, the fact is that fewer students are now applying to dental schools than in the years since 1975. The annual number of applicants has declined by more than 66 percent since 1975, with the largest decline among students from the middle class, according to a study made by the A.D.A. Council on Dental Education in 1989. A steady decrease in all areas of graduate school enrollment has paralleled this decrease in dental school applicants. Funds in 1981 and 1982 were severely limited, with the availability of National Guaranteed Student Loans decreasing steadily, according to the A.D.A. Division of Educational Measurements.

The academic course load in dental school has been mentioned as being too heavy for a student to consider working while in dental school. Let's look at the usual courses required. The majority of dental schools are four-year courses of study, although one dental school is on a five-year program and two are on three-year programs. It is unlikely that the dental school will allow advanced placement or placing out of certain classes even though a student may be quite proficient in a course. The first year of study in a four-year program will probably require the following courses:

Fall Term:

Course	Clock Hours	Credit Hours
Community Dentistry	54	2

Course:	Clock Hours	Credit Hours
Gross Anatomy	176	8
Orthodontics	15	1
Occlusion	40	2
Oral Pathology	14	1
Dental Anatomy	52	3
General Histology	120	5
	471	22

Winter Term:

Course:	Clock Hours	Credit Hours
Elective	45	3
Physiology	64	4
Craniofacial Growth	15	1
Neuroscience	42	3
Oral Diagnosis	30	2
Community Dentistry	15	1
Occlusion	14	1
Biochemistry	72	5
Preclinical Dentistry	90	4
Oral Biochemistry	16	1
Oral Histology	48	2
Emergency Treatment	15	1
Periodontics	45	2
	511	30

The second year of study will include:

Fall Term:

Course:	Clock Hours	Credit Hours
Oral Physiology	15	1
Oral Diagnosis	15	1
Oral Diagnosis Clinic	18	1
Community Dentistry	15	1
Occlusion	15	1
Occlusion Laboratory	33	1
Dental Materials	30	2
Preclinical Dentistry	224	9
Pathology Lecture	45	3
Pathology Laboratory	135	3
Periodontic Clinic	16	¾
	561	23¾

Winter Term:

Course:	Clock Hours	Credit Hours
Elective	45	3
Internal Medicine	15	1
Oral Diagnosis Clinic	27	1
Microbiology	75	4
Oral Physiology	8	½
Dental Materials	30	2
Crown and Bridge	15	1
Preclinical Dentistry	211	9
Oral Pathology	45	3
Oral Pathology Lab	30	1
Anesthesia	21	1½
Pedodontics	15	1
Periodontics	15	1
Periodontics Clinic	15	¾
	567	29¾

The third year of study will cover:

Fall Term:

Course:	Clock Hours	Credit Hours
Pharmacology	45	3
Head and Neck Anatomy	42	2
Oral Diagnosis	15	1
Community Dentistry	30	2
Occlusion	8	½
Endodontics	15	1
Crown and Bridge	15	1
Complete Denture	15	1
Operative Dentistry	15	1
Oral Surgery	8	½
Pedodontics	15	1
Periodontics	15	1
Clinical Conference	10	0
Operative Dentistry Clinic	60	3
Periodontics Clinic	30	1½
Oral Diagnosis Clinic	24	1
Hospital Dentistry	24	1
Endodontics Clinic	42	2

	Clock Hours	Credit Hours
Crown and Bridge Clinic	42	2
Orthodontics Clinic	36	1½
	508	27½

Winter Term:

Course:	Clock Hours	Credit Hours
Elective	45	3
Oral Microbiology	30	2
Community Dentistry	30	2
Cell Biology	15	1
Nutrition	15	1
Partial Denture	15	1
Operative Dentistry Clinic	60	3
Oral Surgery	30	2
Pedodontics	15	1
Periodontics	15	1
Periodontics Clinic	30	1½
Orthodontics	30	2
Clinic Conferences	10	0
Oral Surgery Clinic	24	1
Pedodontics Clinic	24	1
Complete Denture Clinic	42	2
Partial Denture Clinic	42	2
Community Practice	16	¾
Occlusion Clinic	18	1
	507	27¾

There will probably be a summer course requirement between the junior and senior year of dental school, and the courses covered will be:

Course:	Clock Hours	Credit Hours
Elective	45	3
Occlusion	15	1
Dental Materials	15	1
Pedodontics	15	1
Clinical Conferences	15	0
Occlusion Clinic	24	1
Endodontics Clinic	48	2

Hospital Dentistry	32	1½
Complete Denture Clinic	104	5
Operative Dentistry Clinic	180	9
Oral Surgery Clinic	72	3
Orthodontics Clinic	30	1½
Community Practice	40	2¼
	457	22¼

The final and fourth year of study will cover:

Fall Term:

Course:	Clock Hours	Credit Hours
Elective	45	3
Community Dentistry	30	2
Occlusion	15	1
Oral Pathology	15	1
Complete Denture	15	1
Partial Denture	15	1
Oral Surgery	15	1
Oral Pharmacology	30	2
Clinical Conferences	15	0
Oral Diagnosis Clinic	72	3
Crown and Bridge Clinic	104	5
Partial Denture Clinic	104	5
Pedodontics Clinic	72	3
Periodontics Clinic	120	6
	539	27¾

Winter Term:

Course:	Clock Hours	Credit Hours
Elective	45	3
Oral Pathology	15	1
Community Dentistry	30	2
Occlusion	15	1
Endodontics	15	1
Clinical Conferences	10	0
Clinical Class Conferences	15	0
Completion of Clinics	334	15¾
	494	24¾

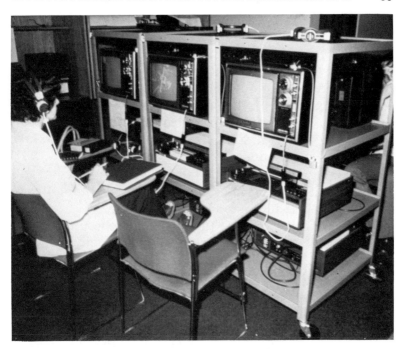

Students have the opportunity to review dental instructional television tapes as often as necessary in the audio-visual-computer center (University of Michigan School of Dentistry, Photographic Department).

During the fourth year, it is not unusual for students to require more than the 494 clock hours to complete clinical assignments, and most schools recognize this. Therefore, 494 clock hours are assigned, but the majority of students have to put in about 550 clock hours in order to complete clinical requirements by graduation day.

As you can see, there is rarely a student who is too well prepared for the rigors of professional school. That is why I and all the other adults around are continuously exhorting the young student to put forth his or her best effort and strive his or her hardest to achieve excellence. These diligent habits will stand the student in good stead as a dental student and as a dentist.

One common complaint heard from dental students is the absence of significant clinical time with patients in the first two years of dental school. The first two years are heavily devoted to academic, dental, medical, and scientific study in preparation for dealing with actual patients. However, recognition of this rationale does not satisfy the enthusiasm of the anxious student. Some dental schools are placing first-year students in clinical situations to take advantage of this understandable enthusiasm.

Let's take a few minutes to speak with some dental students to find out their impressions of dental school. Please keep in mind that these are opinions only.

What are some reasons these students chose dentistry? One frequent answer was that a parent, usually a father, was a dentist. Several women students had been hygienists or nurses and had become disenchanted with those fields. One student had thoroughly examined his aptitudes and felt that dentistry suited him because of his abilities.

Some of the students did express doubts about their decision to go to dental school. One cited the failing economy, stating that they cannot expect to make the kind of money in the future that dentists have made in the past. Another said that if he had known dental school was going to be so hard, he would have gone to medical school instead. By and large, most of the students were satisfied with the choice to enter dental school and would make it again.

Surprisingly, many students had little or no idea what dentistry was all about before entering dental school.

When asked what was the worst thing about dental school for them, many students gave a response quite different from that of practicing dentists: lack of free time. Also, no control over one's time was seen as a negative aspect of dental school. Others were astonished at the amount of study required, to the exclusion of many other important things in their lives. One young student felt that dental school had contributed to her early divorce. Another said, "The cost in personal relationships, finances, and time is enormous." Another said, "I have no outside life. Dental school takes all my time." Still another cited the constant pressure and overwhelming academic load as stressful. One student said, "All the couples we socialize with are dental students or young dentists," and, "Dental school is my whole life right now—unfortunately." Another complained about the financial strain: "I have no money to do anything, even if I could find the time." Finally, a student felt that his mother's grave illness was not given the attention it warranted because he could not get away from dental school to be at her side; he wonders if the guilt from a decision that he felt was forced upon him will always remain with him.

One student described a problem with the manual aspects of dentistry, early in dental school.

Some were afraid that all their long years of study would not pay off because they had heard rumors about an over-supply of dentists, the commercialization of dentistry, and increased government regulation.

Another complaint was that the dental school faculty did not treat the students fairly. Some of the pressure in dental school was arbitrary and not necessary, they said.

There were many positive things about dental school for these students. There were certain professors under whose tutelage the students flourished. They felt lucky to be in on the latest in dental research, perhaps even before practicing dentists learned about certain findings.

The students formed close bonds with other students, bonds that they believe will last a lifetime. They were happy to be exposed to many different types of people, from many parts of the country and of the world. They found it challenging to work with the varied professors.

Many students cited the interaction with the patients as the most positive aspect of dental school. "The patients

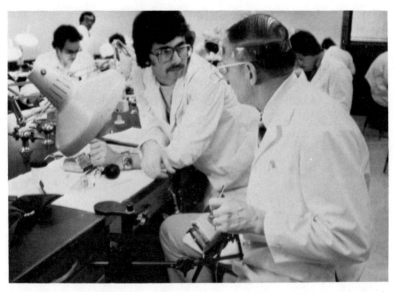

Professors take a personal interest and pride in making difficult procedures understandable to the individual dental student (University of Michigan School of Dentistry, Photographic Department).

make it all worthwhile," was a common comment. They enthusiastically felt that they would really be able to help people when they graduated. Others took enormous pride in the work itself. They had never realized they were capable of such intricate procedures. They felt that they were accomplishing much and making greater strides in their personal development; a new enhancement of their self-image was noticed.

Others cited the many avenues that will be open to them once they graduate and are licensed. A student said, "I will go into pathology because I have found that I am better with my head than my hands. I am glad that option is open to me." One woman was fascinated to discover that dentistry was "so interesting." Even those who were somewhat overwhelmed by the academic workload found dental school stimulating mentally, manually, and psychologically.

One student commented that financial aid was fairly

easy to obtain, but that the eventual repayment of student loans was worrisome, something to fret over later.

Some studens said they had come to "love the work itself" and no other reason was needed to go into dentistry. For some, dental school was a "great experience." Most believed that they would flourish once dental school was behind them.

It behooves the young person to consider his or her career choice seriously; what do YOU want from your life's work?

Now that the young person has examined the profession thoroughly and the course of study required has been reviewed, let us review what steps will be required in order finally to become a dentist. First, he or she will have to graduate from an accredited high school with a high level of achievement in the college-prep classes and take the college boards. Then he or she will complete the undergraduate requirements for the predental course of study. Next the student will take the Dental Aptitude Test and will apply to the schools of his or her choice. The student who is likely to be seriously considered for a place in the freshman class will be granted an interview with the admissions committee. Upon admission, he or she will apply him or herself to the rigors of the dental school education. Thereafter, the state licensing exam will be taken, and the student will finally be able to begin his or her career. What are these tests like, the Dental Aptitude Test and the licensing examination?

If the student will write to the A.D.A. (211 East Chicago Avenue, Chicago, IL 60611) and request material on the Dental Aptitude Test (D.A.T.) or will visit the library and look up books about the test, he or she can find specific answers to questions of personal importance. There are sample D.A.T.'s that the student can purchase and study in privacy. In general, this test is given twice a year, in April and October. The deadline for application is one month prior to the test date, and the fee for 1986-87 was $50; this fee includes the submission of scores to five dental schools and a personal copy to the test-taker. Other transcripts of the scores will be sent out at a charge of $4 each. Applicants are allowed to take the D.A.T. four times; however, test scores for all tests taken will be sent to the five requested dental schools. About 30 percent of predental students do retake the D.A.T. at least twice.[5]

The test itself is about six hours long, with a break for lunch. The four areas examined are:

1. Reading comprehension in dental and basic sciences.
2. Quantitative ability to include math problems in algebra, geometry, and calculus.
3. Perceptual ability to include two- and three-dimensional problem-solving, cubic arrangements, line and angle sequences, multiple angles and circles, three-dimensional problems to include aerial view, side view, and perspective drawings and puzzles, keyhold problems and folding boxes. This portion of the test has taken the place of the famous chalk-carving exercise of the recent past.
4. Survey of the natural sciences, to include biology, general chemistry, and organic chemistry.
   A. Biology—Origin of life, cell metabolism, enzymes, thermodynamics, organelle structure and function, biological organization of major taxa using the five kingdom system, the structure and function of the integumentary, skeletal, muscular, circulatory, immunological, digestive, respiratory, urinary, nervous, endocrine, and reproductive systems, embryology and development, Mendelian inheritance, genetics, meiosis, natural selection, population genetics, speciation, ecology, and animal and social behavior.

[5]American Dental Association, "Dental Admission Testing Program, 1982-1983."

B. General chemistry—Stoichiometry, gases, acids and bases, chemical equilibrium, thermodynamics, thermochemistry, kinetics, oxidation-reduction reactions, atomic and molecular structure, periodic properties, and nuclear reactions.
C. Organic chemistry—Bonding mechanisms, chemical and physical properties of molecules, organic analysis, stereochemistry, nomenclature, reaction of the major functional groups, acid-base chemistry, equilibria, aromatic and synthesis.

A time breakdown shows that thirty-five minutes are spent on biology, fifty-five minutes on chemistry, sixty minutes on reading comprehension, twenty-five minutes on synonyms, fifty minutes on math, twenty-five minutes on verbal analogies, fifteen minutes on line rankings, thirty minutes on spatial relations, fifteen minutes on angle comparisons, and thirty minutes on cubic problems.

Typical Schedule of the D.A.T.

9:00 a.m.—10:30 a.m.	Survey of the Natural Sciences
10:40 a.m.—11:40 a.m.	Reading Comprehension
11:15 a.m.—12:20 p.m.	2-D Perceptual Ability
12:15 p.m.— 1:15 p.m.	Lunch
1:15 p.m.— 2:15 p.m.	Scholastic Ability
2:25 p.m.— 2:55 p.m.	3-D Perceptual Ability

No one is expected to know all the answers on the D.A.T., and there is no penalty for guessing. So do not leave any blank spaces on the answer sheet. Take an accurate watch with you to the test and four or five of the required number two pencils along with the identification card that will be mailed to you. Nothing else is allowed in the testing center. Do not, under any circumstances, be tempted to cheat. The patterns of all test answers are checked by computer and are matched to the seating arrangement for the day; when the computer detects cheating, the applicant's test is voided and a report is sent to all dental schools in the U.S. and Canada. The applicant is then barred from taking the D.A.T. for a period of time, usually one year. Do not hesitate to safeguard your answers.

How are the scores reported to the dental schools? The report includes a guide for interpretation of D.A.T. scores because the coded scores are on a scale from 1 to 9, with 9 being the highest score. These coded scores make it easier for dental schools to compare the performances of all applicants. The coded scores are arrived at by the percentage of applicants receiving a certain score out of 100 percent; the coded score of 4 is the mean and represents that score out of 100 percent that the largest number of students received.

Coded Score	% Receiving That Score	Percentile Equivalent
9	1.1%	98.9 – 99.9
8	2.8%	97.0 – 98.8
7	6.6%	90.0 – 96.0
6	12.1%	78.0 – 89.0
5	17.5%	61.0 – 77.0
4	19.8%	40.0 – 60.0
3	17.5%	23.0 – 39.0
2	12.1%	11.0 – 22.0
1	6.6%	4.0 – 10.0
0	2.8%	1.2 – 3.0
–1	1.1%	0.0 – 1.1

Any score less than four would indicate that the student should study to improve that ability and retake the D.A.T. However, it is not necessary to try to achieve nines in every category; the percentile equivalents show that a seven is actually a high score of 96.0 percent. It's just that a few test-takers were able to achieve a score higher than that.

Young people ask if they should prepare for the D.A.T. Of course, the answer is "yes." Some of the material covered may have been taken by the applicant in college as long as two or three years earlier. The applicant should go about preparing him or herself rationally. Begin by concentrating on areas of known weakness. If the student knows math is a weak area, that is where he or she should spend most of the review time. Next, consider the subjects that were taken the longest time ago. Review all subjects at least minimally by going through the textbooks currently used at the college. There is no need to purchase new textbooks, since the school library will have them. Certainly, it would be impossible to read all the textbooks, and that is not necessary; reread only those chapters or pages that seem unfamiliar to you. Do not attempt to cram on the day before the D.A.T. If at all possible, engage in an activity that is totally divorced from the academic world, preferably a sporting or exercising activity. A day swimming and sailing at the beach would be excellent, but it's pretty cold in April and October in the northern climates. Eat properly and consume no alcohol or pharmaceuticals for at least twenty-four hours prior to the test. A physically tiring day should allow you to get to bed early for a good night's sleep.

Rise at least two hours prior to the exam; if you have to travel, allow plenty of time for the commute. Arriving in a nervous state of stress will lower one's concentrating ability. Do not drink over two cups of coffee prior to or during the exam. It may seem impossible, but try to relax; relaxing is your best assurance of doing well. Remember, at least 30 percent retake the D.A.T. Wouldn't it be fantastic to obtain all nines the first time around? But let's face it: all nines is a fantasy. Even if you do have to retake the test, you'll be out the $50 testing fee, another testing day, and more specific study time. More important, put this experience into perspective: most of the other test-takers are in the same boat as you, and most important, you should be able to leave under your own power, with a clear head and a clear conscience. The D.A.T. is not the beginning or the end of the world.

After about six weeks the D.A.T. scores are sent to the dental schools you have indicated. Your college transcripts should already be there, along with your application. Make and keep photocopies of all your correspondence with the school. Letters do get lost in the mail, and you can make a strong case for yourself if you've had the foresight to keep dated photocopies along with a journal of significant dates. There was one applicant whose parents had taken an official-looking letter from a dental school to her at her summer job. Together, they discovered that the student had been accepted for a place in the autumn freshman class. After work, the student placed the letter on the dashboard and drove home; on the expressway, a crosswind was set up when she rolled down all the windows to alleviate the stifling heat. A gust picked up the letter and whisked it right out of the car. The student drove home, practically in tears, and told her mother what had happened. Together, they returned to the site on the expressway and searched up and down the highway for the letter until a police officer arrived and practically had to drag them away. No trace of the acceptance letter was ever found. The applicant phoned the dental school, and the secretary agreed to send her a copy of the original letter. Can you imagine the good-natured laughter that filled the secretary's office as she related the student's dilemma? Things stranger than this happen all the time, and it is so much better to take a few simple precautions and to be prepared for life's unexpected problems.

On the dental school application itself, answer all questions honestly, including any answers that may be less than complimentary. You can attach a sheet explaining why a certain area of your application is less than ideal. There are very few young people (or old people, for that matter) who cruise through life without a mistake. More important is what did you do to rectify the situation and what have you learned from it? If possible, type the application, but at the very least, use black or dark blue ink and print clearly. You'd be surprised how many young adults resort to the sixth-grade antics of trying to impress others with unique penmanship. The dental school is not interested in your cleverness; they are interested in efficiency and concise and clear presentations.

In the typed biographical sketch attached to the application, you can follow this guide:

1. In the letterhead, include your name, address, phone number, date of the application, and your birthdate.
2. Begin by briefly stating where you were born, and where you have lived.
3. Name all the schools you have attended by years, location, and date. If you attended a special training session or a special school, mention that also. For example, while in high school, did you take part in a creative writing workshop at a nearby college? Did you attend a special high school where students were admitted according to ability? Or perhaps you made an error in judgment in high school and did not take the college-prep course; what have you done in the recent past to remedy that? Perhaps you've since completed junior college work and college work at a high level of proficiency that shows you are capable of excellence.
4. Very briefly, sketch your mother's and father's occupations and background. There is no reason to believe that your parents' lives will affect your chance of being accepted into dental school; each candidate is judged on his or her own record. How-

ever, it is likely that sons and daughters of professionals may have a better understanding of what will be expected of them in their training and professional life.

5. You may include your racial or ethnic background, if you like.
6. List any honors you have received academically.
7. Explain your involvement in extracurricular activities and any awards you've earned in nonacademic endeavors.
8. Describe any church affiliations or church work you've been involved in.
9. List your work experience.
10. Explain any volunteer work you've been doing.
11. What about your hobbies, clubs and organizations you belong to? Do they demonstrate any special talents?
12. Do you have any unique or special experiences you think should be included? Promotions? Travel? Appointments? Publications?
13. What about your military experience? More than a few young people have entered the military fresh out of high school and been assigned and trained as a dental assistant, thereby discovering that they love the field. These young people then have returned to college to complete the predental requirements. The admissions committee needs to know this.
14. What is your marital status and how many children do you have? How will they be cared for? What does your spouse think about your going to a professional school?
15. Why do you think dentistry is the career for you?
16. What are your future plans and ambitions?
17. Attach at least three letters of recommendation, and include the names, positions, addresses, and telephone numbers of the persons writing the letters.

18. Attach a recent, excellent photograph of yourself. It's hard to believe that many applicants actually send a snapshot of themselves at the beach, or when they wore glasses, had a six-inch beard, and were brunette instead of blond.

After the dental school has received your D.A.T. scores, your transcripts, and your application, they will grant you an interview if your chances of being accepted are good.

You must phone the dental school yourself and arrange the interview appointment yourself; do not ask your parents or your spouse to do this for you. Of course, they may take messages while you are out, but you must always call back in person to verify the message. Make sure you use standard business courtesy and identify yourself immediately when you call, and state the reason for your call.

For the interview, dress nicely and conservatively, as if you were going to a church service. Young men and women should wear suits whenever possible, even if the interview takes place in the hot summer. Women should wear hose and close-toed shoes regardless of how great their tan is. The hair should be neat and clean, but not necessarily pulled back. Beards should be neatly trimmed and combed. If you need glasses, wear them so that you're not continuously squinting. Do not fidget or play with your clothes, hair, or glasses while at the interview. Take with you copies of the correspondence with the school, a copy of the school's catalogue, and a small notebook with questions you'd like to ask; place all these loose papers in a briefcase. YOU are being interviewed, so it is up to you to make sure you're there on time, and you take the first step in introducing yourself to the interviewer. Many interviewees do take their parents or spouse with them, and the dental schools do not frown on this. The spouse or parents must realize, however, that they will not be sitting in on the interview, and they must excuse themselves to look around the building or campus after five minutes of small talk with the administrator who has greeted them. If the school offers them a guided tour of the dental school, that is nice, but the parents or spouse should not expect it. There is no advantage or disadvantage to the applicant who takes along spouse or parents, and it is certainly understandable that these important people in the applicant's life are interested and enthusiastic about the career he or she is about to embark upon.

The interview will last from fifteen to thirty minutes. A clear and concise application and autobiographic sketch will shorten the procedure. Usually, three or four members of the admissions committee will be present, but sometimes only one interviewer is available. Before the interview, be sure to get the titles of the committee members correct. Do not call a doctor "Miss," and do not call a dean "Mister." Pronounce the names of the committee members correctly; if one of the names is unusual, it is perfectly acceptable to ask at the beginning of the interview, "Do I have the pronunciation of your name right?" Be as truthful and honest as possible in your answers to questions. Do not avoid any questions by beating around the bush or running off at a tangent. It is perfectly acceptable to say, "I'm sorry, I do not know the answer to that," or "I'd have to think about that a long time before I could answer." Also, when you are asked to explain something on your application, do not criticize or condemn your past teachers or employers. The admissions committee does not care that you did not like a certain teacher or that you did not get along with your boss. They know that you'll have to be able to work with many people in dental school whom you may not particularly like, and that there will be many people in the practice of dentistry whose personalities you do not appreciate; you will nevertheless be expected to get along and perform excellently.

It is natural to be nervous at this interview, but do not

under any circumstances use alcohol or pharmaceuticals to calm yourself. That only makes you appear goofy, and nervous is a better appearance than foolish. Smile when appropriate, but do not giggle or laugh raucously or overlong. Do not try to dominate the interview with your sparkling wit or great sense of humor. Speak clearly and evenly, without little coughs or "ah's," and not too fast. Look straight at the questioner during the question and while you are answering; do not interrupt the other speakers under any circumstances. Here are some questions that may be asked of you:

1. When and why did you first become interested in dentistry?
2. Who has urged you to go into dentistry?
3. What is there about dentistry that you think you'd enjoy? On what experience do you base this?
4. What do your spouse and/or parents think about your attending dental school?
5. What made you choose this school?
6. How do you plan to finance the cost of a dental education?
7. Why did you drop this course?
8. Why did you change colleges?
9. Why didn't you take college-prep when you were in high school?
10. Why did you get such a low grade in this course?
11. Why did you take a semester off?
12. What was the most difficult part of the D.A.T. for you?
13. Why did you take the D.A.T. three times?
14. Explain this unusual experience you had.
15. If you are not accepted in dental school, what are your contingency plans?
16. How do you think you measure up to the other members of the first-year dental class?

17. Why are you changing careers? Do you think your age will make a difference in your performance?

When the interviewers are satisfied, they will ask if you have any questions. Here are a few appropriate queries, and you may add your own to it. But do not take more than ten minutes with your list:

1. Is there a combined degree program at this school?
2. How much off-campus experience is offered to the dental student?
3. What is the average clinic size? What is the ratio of students to faculty in the clinic?
4. When does the student first begin clinical experience?
5. Is the patient flow adequate?
6. Do students ever get the chance to work with a dental assistant?
7. Are summer jobs available at the dental school, and is priority given to dental students when hiring?

At the end of the interview, use common politeness and say, "It was nice to meet you, Dr. X, Dr. Y, and Dr. Z. Thank you for your time." Because you have adequately prepared yourself, you will have been able to present your true personality in a complimentary light. Enjoy the rest of the day with your spouse or parents exploring the school and campus.

Let's suppose that you are rejected in spite of your best efforts. Remember, there are many more applicants than spaces available in the first-year class, so some qualified applicants will be rejected. By all means, write a polite note to the admissions committees of the schools you applied to and ask them if there was a specific area of weakness that caused your rejection. You can and should take steps to improve that area. You may retake the D.A.T. up to four times, and you can reapply next year to the same dental schools or to others. With all this information on hand, approach your predental counselor for advice. Only 92 percent of the entering freshman class are expected to graduate from dental school, so errors in judgment are made by admissions committees as well as by applicants. Perhaps you would be better off to pursue another career in a related health field, or you might even be happier in a field totally apart from health. It would be much more disastrous to discover this after four expensive years of dental school, passing the state boards, and practicing for several years, than to face the reality at this point in your life.

The state boards themselves have generated much stress for recent graduates and older dentists alike. There is no national licensure for dentists now, and few states have reciprocal licensing agreements. This means that a dentist cannot practice in a state until he or she has met that state's requirements. The requirements differ from state to state, so a dentist's mobility can be severely hampered if he or she decides to move. An unfortunate situation arose for a forty-eight-year-old dentist whose wife developed a health problem. After many medical tests, examinations, and referrals, it was determined that she needed both a change in climate and special treatments available at only a few clinics. The couple decided to move to a state where there was such a clinic and where the climate was better. While his wife was undergoing therapy, the dentist was faced with difficulties he had not anticipated; he had to take the state board examination in dentistry four times before he passed—this after he had practiced dentistry for twenty-three years. Without question, he had to obtain this license, since his working as a dentist was to support himself, his wife, and their youngest son, a teenager. In addition, he had huge medical expenses to meet. Imagine the awful stress and tension he underwent as he studied and restudied the dental texts into the wee hours of the night, hoping and praying to pass the boards.

Also, the fee to take the state boards needs to be considered; this fee varies from state to state. Added to that is the cost of materials and travel and providing patients. If a dentist has to take the state boards three or four times, it can be quite money-, time-, and psyche-consuming. Many organizations and dentists are addressing the licensing issue, but a resolution seems a long way off.

As an example of what to expect on a state board, the North East Regional Board Examination will be cited. This exam does cover thirteen states. Each year the exam is conducted three times: the third week of May, the third week of August, and the third week of December. The purpose is to test the clinical competence of candidates for licensure in dentistry and in dental hygiene, and the two examinations are run concurrently. There is a five-part series of tests in dentistry and a two-part series in dental hygiene. The examination includes objective and clinical performance; the objective portion is corrected by computer, and the clinical portion is judged by examiners. A score of less than 75 percent in any part is considered a failing grade. The five sections are as follows:

1. The section on Diagnosis, Oral Medicine, and Radiology is an objective, multiple-choice written test. There is a presentation of a number of patients simulated by the projection of color transparencies or radiographs with pertinent histories. Candidates are expected to identify conditions, pathologies, and accepted outlines of treatment.
2. A second section requires the candidate to prepare a comprehensive treatment plan for patients. Photographs of the patient's casts and radiographs are supplied along with the case history. Candidates also are required to evaluate a series of color slides and radiographs of other clinical cases and on the basis of short case histories select the diagnosis and

treatment plan for each in a multiple-choice examination.

3. A third portion of the exam is Restorative Dentistry. The candidate selects one procedure from each of two types and must then complete the two procedures within a time limit on a live patient. Included among the restorations in the two categories of procedures are: gold foil, gold inlay/onlay, silver amalgam, 3/4 and full cast gold crowns.

4. A fourth section of the examination on Periodontics requires certain routine procedures with a live patient within a certain time limit.

5. The final section of the test, on Prosthetic Dentistry, consists of a complete denture exercise requiring certain procedures with a live patient.

The examination takes place over a three-day period, 8:00 a.m. to 5:00 p.m., with an hour for lunch. The candidate is required to supply all medications, medicaments, supplies, sundries, instruments, and patients. In addition, two eight-hour tests called the National Boards are given prior to one's application for the N.E.R.B.: first at the end of the sophomore year and then four months prior to the N.E.R.B., usually in December of the senior year. These are objective, multiple-choice examinations. Some states do not require the National Board tests to be taken, although the majority of states do.

The cost for the N.E.R.B. was $530 in 1987. In addition, most states charge a separate licensing fee, the amount of which varies from state to state. The applicants wait about six to eight weeks before the results are mailed to them, and each applicant is allowed to retake the exam as many times as necessary within a five-year period, although evidence of remedial education must be submitted if the candidate fails more than two times.

Most state board examinations are similar to this; relicensure may be annual and biennial. Continuing education is a prerequisite for relicensure in eleven states. However, a particular state should be contacted to find out the precise requirements for licensure to practice dentistry in that state.

As soon as the state boards are passed, the young dentist can begin to treat patients in a clinic or in his or her own practice; however, many dentists opt to specialize at this point. The specialties listed in Chapter I are the only specialties recognized by the A.D.A. and by the fifty states. They require adherence to a specific training program at an accredited dental school and residency programs associated with the dental schools or with accredited hospitals. The cost and time requirements of specialization vary, but a range of expenses in 1989 was $3,000 per semester for a resident and up to $10,000 for a nonresident. Most programs are two-year programs, with the exception of oral/maxillofacial surgery, which is a three-year program at most institutions. The specialist must then pass another set of board examinations in his or her state before qualifying as a specialist. In addition, great prestige and privilege can be obtained by becoming a Diplomate or Fellow of the specialty, and another rigorous examination is associated with that. Some specialists also need to obtain hospital privileges, since many of the procedures they will perform have to be done in a hospital setting.

When a dentist or specialist is in practice, his or her education is still not complete. Some states require postgraduate education for relicensure and some do not. Diplomate or Fellow status requires a certain number of postgraduate hours to be taken every year. All conscientious dentists make an effort to attend continuing education classes in order to assure that their patients are afforded the latest and most sophisticated treatment available. The cost of these classes varies, but most dentists find the courses well worth the expense. A dental career means a commitment to lifelong learning and improvement: "If you live to learn, you'll learn to live."

V

I couldn't believe it when my daughter came running into the house crying because her mouth was bleeding. I mopped up the mess with a clean washcloth and discovered that a tooth was missing. I remembered a dentist speaking at a P.T.A. meeting about knocked-out teeth, so I ran over to the baseball diamond to look for it. It was behind second base, covered with dirt. I did not wash it off, but dropped it into a bowl of warm tap water, called our family dentist, and rushed Jennifer over to his office.

Jennifer was not very well behaved, but Dr. Jim, a family friend, was able to calm her enough to give her an injection. Then he reinserted the tooth into the socket and wired it in place. He placed her on antibiotics. Her lip swelled up pretty big, but she healed up in ten days. Dr. Jim removed the wires in six weeks and tested the tooth. It was dead, and the dentist sent us to a specialist, an endodontist, for root canal treatment. This Dr. Janet Snow was very businesslike and asked me to leave the room while she treated Jennifer. Of course, Jennifer was very well-behaved there since there was no pain, and Dr. Snow explained everything thoroughly. Those treatments took three visits.

As Dr. Snow had explained it sometimes happens, the tooth darkened to a gray color when Jennifer was fifteen and very self-conscious. Dr. Jim explained that there was a simple procedure whereby the tooth could be bleached back to its normal color, and that Jennifer may have to have a crown placed at a later date.

79

The bleaching was a success, and Janet is looking forward to going to the prom in this, her junior year in high school.

Mrs. Wallace has four other children and is one level-headed lady. Her quick thinking saved Jennifer's tooth and so averted the more extensive treatments involved in bridgework. She cannot remember the name of the dentist who spoke at that P.T.A. meeting so long ago, but every time Jennifer flashes that beautiful smile, she thinks of him, Dr. Jim, and the aloof Dr. Snow.

Chapter V

What to Do With Your DDS?

The newly graduated dentist can look forward to a rich and rewarding life; the career opportunities opening up to him or her are wide and varied. He or she can choose from widely divergent routes: establish a private practice; purchase a practice; enter an associateship; buy into an established practice over a period of years; incorporate his or her practice; enter a career in government service; enter a lifetime of teaching or research; work for a commercial dental chain; enter dental missionary work; or become an administrator in the dental field.

Once the state board examinations have been passed, the dentist is entitled to establish his or her own practice; in 1987, 91 percent of the practicing dentists were in private practice. The expense of setting up a practice varies, but the most basic office begins at $75,000 and the cost can go as high as $250,000. As pointed out in Chapter IV, the average debt of a graduating dentist in 1990 was $45,000. Coming up with an additional $70,000 or more would be difficult for anyone who is not independently wealthy.

Many young dentists purchase the practice of a retiring dentist. Included in the purchase price are the equipment, supplies, furnishings, and goodwill of the retiring dentist. There are standard formulas for valuing the equipment, supplies, and furnishings, but the goodwill is a point of much debate. A young dentist can expect to pay between $50,000 and $300,000 to buy out an established dentist.

Obviously, the higher the price, the greater the income the young dentist can expect to receive from the practice. Also, a lesser price could reflect very old equipment and dated supplies and furnishings. Many young dentists anticipate using the older equipment just long enough to get the practice going, and they plan later to procure another loan to refurbish the office.

Some dentists buy into an existing practice. The dentist who owns the practice is not interested in retiring but is willing to take on a partner. Like any business, the cost depends on the success of the particular practice. Again, the young dentist will be purchasing some goodwill, since he or she will benefit from the older dentist's reputation and established patient list. The cost can vary from $30,000 to $150,000, and this purchase price automatically puts the young dentist on an equal standing with the older dentist. The new dentist can expect to influence office policy and can challenge policy if he or she sees the need. Also, the new dentist now has the right to the benefits offered to partners in the practice.

These costs do not include a building, in most cases. Indeed, most dentists do not even consider owning a building until they are out of dental school for quite a number of years. Many dentists never wish to own and maintain a building.

For the dentist with few resources and without the likelihood of obtaining a substantial loan, a common means of entering private practice is an associateship. In essence, the young dentist works in the established dentist's office and receives a certain percentage of the collections for his or her efforts. For example, the associate may receive 40 to 50 percent of the fees collected from the patients he or she treats. The established dentist keeps the other percentage to cover overhead, pays the young dentist on a biweekly or monthly basis, and does not provide any benefits or even take out the necessary taxes. In fact, some dentists associate in two or three offices, and the dollar amount the young dentist receives each pay period varies greatly. For example, December is a very low month for collections in most dental offices, and this is the month when the associate will therefore receive the least amount of pay.

The associate has virtually no responsibility or say in running the office or in challenging established policy. For example, if the office has a policy of not treating relatives, the younger dentist has to abide by this whether or not he or she agrees with it. Also, there is little or no protection for the associate, especially if no agreement has been signed. It is unusual for an established dentist purposely to set out to cheat an associate; more likely is that the dentist may decide to let the associate go for any reason, and the young dentist has no recourse except to go. Some younger dentists leave an associateship in a year or two because the established dentist and the office personnel will not relinquish any authority; the receptionists, assistants, or hygienists may have been employed by the older dentist for ten or twenty years. Dentists are often described as being highly individualistic, and so it is easy to understand that a personality conflict may occur.

However, the younger dentist also has virtually no responsibility in running the practice and so does not have to face the headaches of coordinating all the facets of a business. If an assistant is ill, it is the older dentist who has to find a temporary replacement; it is the older dentist who is responsible for meeting the tax liability of the business; it is the older dentist who has to say "no" to the personnel's requests for raises; it is the older dentist who has to make certain the equipment is maintained; it is the older dentist who has to contact the landlord when building maintenance is not up to par; it is the older dentist who is paid last, after all the other bills have been paid; it is the older dentist who has to deal with severe patient-relations problems, even though it may have been the associate who erred. In other words, it is the older dentist who has to take the headaches home every night and weekend. Many young graduates are simply not ready to assume these responsibilities.

Most associateship arrangements work out excellently, depending on the personalities of the dentists involved. The arrangement has been so popular for so long because it fills a need for both parties.

As an owner or a part-owner in a practice, there is no question of "authority." As mentioned before, the dollar cost is substantial. How is a young dentist to acquire these large sums of money? One common way is to "buy into" an established practice. The method is a cross between an outright purchase and an associateship. The young dentist makes a certain down payment, usually a fraction of the agreed-upon total cost. He or she and the older dentist sign a legal document that details all the specifics worked out with a lawyer and a certified public accountant. Basically, this dentist works for a percentage of his or her personal gross, to cover the same percentage that the office carries as an overhead figure. Then more percentage points are subtracted from the dentist's take-home pay for a specific number of years until the remaining debt is paid off, usually five to ten years. Occasionally, the young dentist's earnings far exceed the original expectations, and he or she is able to pay off the debt before the specified date. More likely, the young dentist has a family to think about and all its expenses, and he or she has to take home the maximum amount possible, so the debt can cover quite a period of time. As soon as the new dentist has become a part-owner, by making the down payment, he or she is entitled to the fringe benefits of the practice. Each practice is different, but fringe benefits can include health care insurance and related costs, day-care arrangements, uniforms, business lunches, trips to seminars, and profit-sharing and pension plans. In fact, the dollar amount of take-home pay in a given practice may not be as attractive as the benefit package, but the new dentist may opt for the larger benefits because it suits his or her family situation better than straightforward income. A dentist who establishes his or her own practice will also have the opportunity to obtain these benefits, but it may be years before the young practice can support them.

There is also the question of whether or not a private practice should incorporate. The corporation laws vary from state to state, and a young person interested in corporate law should contact the state government offices to learn the specifics. Generally, licensed doctors in the U.S. are legally allowed to incorporate a clinic or a practice and are covered by the same laws, privileges, and responsibilities that cover any corporation. The dentist may choose to be the only employee in the corporation; or any number of clinicians and personnel may be employed. Are there advantages or disadvantages to incorporation? Any number of arguments can be started and become unending, with experts such as certified public accountants and lawyers on either side. The young dentist needs to know this option is available so that a mistake in his or her particular situation will not be made—a mistake that might be quite costly.

Let me point out that the dental education one receives in U.S. dental schools is second to none. The scientific and clinical training is superb. However, there is virtually no training in the operation of a dental practice and its business aspects. Most new graduates are overwhelmed by the tax, corporate, and business laws governing them and other small businesses. The truth is, many fine clinicians are driven out of practice by this burgeoning bureaucratic maze. Adding to the confusion are the seminars and classes and experts who claim to have all the answers, for a substantial fee, of course. Although this quandary will not be faced until graduation or well after graduation, it will be a difficult decision, and the difficulty should not be underestimated.

For these reasons, including lack of financial resources, lack of business training, and uncertainty, many young dentists seek employment in federal, state, and local government, teaching, research, administrative positions, and commercial dental chains.

The federal government employs about 6,200 dentists in the Public Health Service, the Veterans Administration, and the Armed Forces. The Army, the Navy, and the Air Force operate on a similar basis and a similar pay scale. The geographic coverage of the services is worldwide, and the young dentist may end up in an Alaskan village north of the Arctic Circle or in the heat of the Mideast. The entering dentist's request for a specific location is considered, but it's obvious that he or she will have to go where the assignment is. For the initial enlistment period, there is about an 80 percent match between area of preference and assignment. Some dentists who decide to make government service a career enjoy the transfers and the challenge of new locations and environments. Others cannot take the regimentation and relocating and are relieved to get out after the three-year obligation. Each dentist's personality and situation are unique, and so is his or her response to the services.

In 1976 Congress discontinued military scholarships, grants, or loans for dental students' expenses. In 1980 all dental student scholarships and loan credits based on federal service were phased out until such time as Congress sees a need to reinstate them.

The dentist enters the Public Health Service with the rank of Senior Assistant, the Army with the rank of Captain, the Navy and the Air Force with the rank of Lieutenant, and the Veterans Administration with the title of

Associate. In the Public Health Service and the armed services, there are six levels to which the dentist can rise; in the Veterans Administration, there are nine. At the entry level the dentist can expect to earn $24,000 in basic pay, but there are other benefits as well, including complete health care for the dentist and his or her family, housing or a housing allowance, scheduled bonuses, paid-for trips to seminars, use of cars, supplied uniforms, the P.X., and certain tax benefits (some military benefits are nontaxable). The final figure an entering dentist can earn depends on his or her family size and can be the equivalent of $34,000. Each year of service and each reenlistment can earn the dentist a sizable bonus; the reenlistment is from year to year for a one-year period. There is an attractive retirement policy in the services and an increase in rank and pay for time served. However, all these incentives are subject to approval by Congress, and the fringes can vary over time. Many young people who had no intention of making a career out of federal service decide that there are advantages and rewards in a service career for them.

In the services, it is easy to understand that there is much regimentation. The dentist is required to meet military obligations as well as those of dentistry; these include programs and indoctrinations; lectures and seminars, and possible field duty. This regimentation also covers the dentist's provision of dental services. Most bases have a detailed manual of procedures and how they are to be executed; in fact, sometimes a dentist is told how many patients he or she is supposed to see per day. Twenty-four-hour duty is a real possibility, although most base clinics are arranged on an eight-hour day, with some weekend worktime also scheduled. The supervising officer watches over the dentists, hygienists, and assistants. The supervisor writes progress reports on the personnel, including the dentists, and informs the dentists how to become better army dentists. For many young dentists, to become a supervising officer becomes a goal. For others, the lack of freedom is stifling. Much depends upon the personalities of the dentists involved; but a young dentist just out of dental school is used to regimentation and criticism and is likely to adjust quite well to the clinical situation in government service.

Whether or not the dentist's family will adjust to this life-style is another question. Many a spouse cannot or will not accept the regimentation of life on or near a base. A young person who is married has to discuss all the options thoroughly with his or her spouse rather than just assume that the spouse is willing to go along with whatever is best for the dental student or dentist. Perhaps the spouse would rather carry a debt of $75,000 to $250,000 and forgo certain luxuries to start a private practice than spend several years in a frozen station in Greenland or a jungle in South America. Other spouses may look upon those places as great adventures.

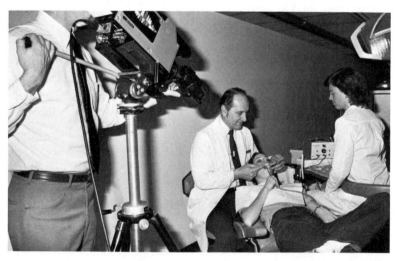

Dr. Robert Lorey, a professor at the University of Michigan, is being photographed for a television instructional tape. The TV tape shows extreme close-ups of the various procedures followed in preparing a tooth to receive a crown (University of Michigan School of Dentistry, Photographic Department).

The National Health Service Corps Scholarship Program offers financial assistance to dental students who agree to serve in the National Public Health Service for a specified time following graduation. According to a survey made in 1986 by the American Association of Dental Schools, 1.7 percent of seniors had National Health Service Corps scholarships.

The young dentist can also consider entering the field of dental education. Many dentists stay on at the school where they were trained, moving through the hierarchy to become full tenured professors. Others go on to other schools in the U.S., Canada, and around the world. Although a student may not realize it, there are philosophical differences in the teaching at the various dental schools, and it is possible to find a school that will suit a particular personality.

The advantage to teaching is not necessarily financial or in the fringe benefits. The instructors and associate, assistant, and full professors do make a good living, and benefits are excellent, but there is a definite ceiling on earnings. Most people who stay on at a dental school do so because they wish to be identified with and to represent the school. There is a certain prestige associated with being a professor. There are also colleagues with whom to share experiences and discoveries; a professorship is not as lonely as a private practice. As in any teaching situation, dental educators must enjoy and like young people. Dental educators must receive a personal, internal reward when that light of understanding flickers across a student's face because of the special knowledge the teacher has shared.

One thing to understand, however, is that the vast majority of professors have no background in education, either theory or methodology. Some find it difficult even to keep the class quiet. This can be very discouraging to the young educator, but the pathway to a professorship simply does not recognize this void. Thus, tried and true teaching methods that a third-grade teacher may have at his or her disposal are not available to the dental educator unless he or she develops them on his or her own or actively seeks out education courses. Even test-writing can be a difficult challenge when one's training in the English language is not superb. Changes in policy and in courses are slow at this level and often have to be approved by numerous committees who are far removed from the everyday problems of dental education.

In the schools there are also regimentation, expectations, and schedules to be considered. The life of the dental educator and his or her family has to revolve around the school's location and functions. The professor also forgoes the daily contact with individual patients; for some, this is the very reason that they enter dental education.

Most dental schools are affiliated with a public school or university. This means that many decisions are made at the state capital that affect the operation of the school. Even federal decisions can have a monumental effect on the dental school. A dental educator may find him or herself in a position of powerlessness in the political arena that will affect his or her dental education career.

Besides educating dental students, a dentist can teach in other schools in the dental field. There are hygiene schools that are separate from the dental schools, as well as schools and training courses for assistants and laboratory technicians. There are even postgraduate schools organized and operated by dentists for other dentists. Some private practitioners combine two careers, one as a dentist in the private office and another as an educator in postgraduate seminars who gives lectures at dental conventions and seminars.

Associated with a career in dental education is work in dental research. The National Institute of Dental Research operates and coordinates laboratories across the nation. A student may become interested as a laboratory assistant, measuring and writing reports. Eventually he or she will begin to design experiments and measurements and finally be able to write a proposal that poses the question of why an experiment is important, why it should be run, and what it is supposed to prove. Many large grants are made to the universities by the federal government and large corporations, and proposals for grants have to be written with professional clarity and precision. Often, the author of such a proposal is called upon to present it in person to a committee before funds are allocated for the research.

Research is not always represented by a thin person in a white coat, steered through life by a thick pair of black-rimmed glasses. Dental research has taken place in Egypt's tombs, in Chile's archeological expeditions, and among native populations in Canada's northernmost reaches. Since diplomatic channels with China have been opened, there has been much exchange and research with Chinese dentists.

Dental researchers also work for corporations and businesses, helping to develop new products and medicines to aid the private dentist and the general population. These dentists are usually spokespersons for the company as well as for the profession. Some dentists even start their own companies if they think they have hit upon an idea or invention that will send tremors throughout the dental world. As in any business in the U.S., there is always the possibility of becoming a millionaire by finding a better way and operating a successful business to market it.

A recent change in the delivery of dental care is the appearance of commercial dental chains similar to the commercial optical chains that have been around for years. Many operate out of large department stores. A comparison can be made between the commercial dental chains and a national fast-food business: all the stores across the country can be easily identified by the sign out in front, the "logo." All the stores are run the same, and the food tastes the same whether it is purchased in Ludington, Michigan, or Phoenix, Arizona, or Anchorage, Alaska. The prices are the same everywhere, as is the service and even the decor of the inside and outside of the building. Everything is standardized, down to the uniforms and hats the workers wear.

Business entrepreneurs, some of whom are dentists, are attempting to do this with dentistry. All the clinics will be operated similarly, using the same products and methods to deliver dental care regardless of location. The fees and hours of service will be the same throughout the country. Dentists will be employees, or they can become franchisees. Since the idea is so new, it is hard to guess what a fair price for a franchise will be. A franchise in the fast-food business costs between $150,000 and $250,000, depending on the success of the national corporation. In 1982 the A.D.A. reported one franchise fee at $20,000, with an additional mandatory purchase of equipment from the corporate headquarters at $125,000; monthly royalties were set at 6 percent of the gross receipts. In exchange for the payments, the franchisor offers a known, national name and business and management expertise and advice.[1]

There are those who salute commercial dental chains as the wave of the future, the greatest thing to happen to dentistry since local anesthetic. Most dentists, however, are extremely leary of the concept and view franchises as a major step backward for the profession, the patients, and the population at large. Can dentistry be standardized? Will a patient with a dental health problem be willing to go to such a place for treatment? Who will assure quality, if not the treating dentist? Should a business entrepreneur with no understanding or training in dentistry make decisions that will affect patients' options and care? Whether or not these philosophical questions can be answered, it seems that there are dentists who are willing either to work in or

---

[1]Beacham, Kendal, "The Delivery of Dental Care," American Dental Association *Journal*, Vol. 105, No. 3, September, 1982.

purchase such a franchise. The private dentist or the young person contemplating private dental practice should not imagine that such commercial dental chains will not draw patients, assistants, and hygienists away from his or her private practice.

Another recent concept is that of the Health Maintenance Organization. These are set up as nonprofit organizations, cooperatives that are owned by the patient-members. The doctors are not paid out of the profits as in a fee-for-service practice, but are paid a set salary, as are all the other employees. The members pay for care on a per capita (per person) basis, usually with a monthly premium. This approach will supposedly result in patients seeking more preventive care rather than waiting for a health problem to arise. The advantages to the dentist who works for such an organization are the elimination of business worries, the many dental colleagues with whom to share experiences and knowledge, the possibility of concentrating on those clinical areas the doctor finds most satisfying, and the presence of other medical specialties under the same roof. The disadvantages are the lack of independence for the individual doctor, the relinquishment of authority, the loss of autonomy, the loss of the patient-doctor relationship, and the inevitable personality frictions among the personnel.

At the opposite end of the spectrum of dentistry are those dentists who enter missionary work. These people do not labor for money, but for modest support from a church or similar organization. There are many philosophies and theories as to why people behave in a certain way. Simply stated, there are those people for whom spiritual and moral values are the primary motivators in their lives. A career in dentistry can be perfectly integrated with this commitment. The poor, needy, and less fortunate of this world are in desperate need of dental services, here in the U.S. and throughout the world. For dentists who cannot make a total commitment to missionary work, there are many patients in our own society who need the special care and talents of a dentist. Mentally and physically handicapped children, foster children, and orphans have no resources of their own and yet are in dire need of all types of dental treatment. If a dentist can give a day a week or even a day a month, there are many groups who will truly appreciate his or her generosity.

In government and private businesses and agencies, there is a need for dental administrators, although this need is limited. Dentists are needed to run the state board examinations, as described in Chapter IV. The state and national dental associations require executive directors, as do clinics and departments in hospital complexes. These administrators and managers do not treat patients or teach students on a one-to-one basis, but are responsible for dealing with larger groups; they formulate and implement policy. Often, these positions require further training beyond dental school; a master's degree in public health or business may be required.

The career possibilities for a dentist are endless. Many avenues are open to the young man or woman who has completed a DDS or DMD program and has proven his or her competence. A young dentist need only be limited by his or her imagination, hard work, conscience, and necessary legal restraints.

VI

I always made certain that my children were taken to the dentist for checkups, but I didn't set a good example. I only went when I thought I had a problem. Now I know that by the time a patient notices the problem, it may be too late.

I am a busy lawyer, and my time is severely limited. But my appearance is very important to me. In fact, my success in the courtroom depends on it, to a degree.

About a year ago, my wife had been complaining about my bad breath and finally made an appointment for me with our dentist. I almost canceled out, but she called my secretary to make sure I got there. The dentist, Dr. Wallinford, didn't realize that I was the father of those nice Dater children he was always treating. He took a health and dental history. One look in my mouth, and he ordered up a full-mouth set of X rays. After his examination, he informed me that I had periodontal disease, a gum disease. His assistant wheeled in a projector, and I watched a tape about the disease. I didn't really believe I had that problem, but Dr. Wallinford assured me that indeed I did have it. He showed me the areas of my gums that were indicative of the problem, and they did look just like the pictures on the tape. He showed the X-ray evidence to me, and I became convinced.

We began some long, hard treatments, but I certainly did not want to lose my teeth. I think, however, that the hardest thing for me was to develop good dental hygiene habits. I had always been too busy to brush, much less floss, my teeth. Dr. Wallinford and his hygienist kept after me, though, in a gentle persuasion.

I now realize that that trip to Dr. Wallinford saved my teeth. As I see my colleagues begin to wear dentures one by one, I am grateful every day that Dr. Wallinford had the patience to stick with it, to persuade me to take care of my teeth.

Mr. Charles E. Dater runs a successful law firm at age fifty. His children are almost all grown up now, and he and his wife are still looking forward to traveling together. They are both still patients of Dr. Wallinford.

Chapter **VI**

Dentistry for Everyone

The level of dental expertise in the United States is far superior to that of any other country in the world. Furthermore, the availability to the general population of this excellent dental care is unrestricted and unsurpassed. However, dentists cannot rest on these laurels, patting themselves on the back, because there are still population groups in the U.S. who are underserved by the dental profession: the racial minorities, the impoverished, the mentally and physically handicapped, the socially disadvantaged, and the very young and the very old. In theory, any and everyone has access to the private practitioner, the primary provider upon whom the health care system in the U.S. is predicated. The utilization of dental care in the general population is based upon the affordability of that care, the attitude of the patient and the doctor, geographic availability, and action by the patient to seek out his or her own care. These four factors can, in fact, limit the delivery of adequate dental care to all people. How these problems can be rectified will depend upon future dentists—those young people who are currently deciding to enter the profession.

The A.D.A., in cooperation with various government agencies, has targeted these problems and has endeavored to find ways to treat them. One approach was to train more minority students as dentists, and Affirmative Action programs took form in the late sixties and during the seventies. Special scholarships were set up in the dental schools by corporations, churches, the government, and the A.D.A.

The approach has had its success. In 1971 there were 6 percent minority dentistry students in the U.S.; in 1979 there were 11 percent.

By increasing the number of minority dentists, several goals have been achieved.

First, it is hoped that the living standard of these dentists and their families will be improved greatly. The above-average income and prestige a dentist can obtain afford the dentist's family a level of security and opportunity not often attained by past generations of minority races. What successful middle-class families have taken for granted for years can be available to the minority dentist and his or her children. The very health of the family of the minority dentist can be excellent since plenty of food will always be available, a healthful home environment can be provided, and the dentist can afford optimal health care for the children. This security gives the children the means, as well as the confidence and expectation, to achieve in school and in any career they eventually choose. It follows that the children in these families will seek a station in life that will also afford *them* a successful, upward-bound family. One goal will have been reached: for minorities to improve their own economic conditions through achievement.

Second, it is believed that minority professionals will provide role models for the youngsters of the nonwhite races. These young students can be more readily exposed to the rigors of the dental profession and can begin to ready themselves in junior high school and high school. A student who waits until age thirty or thirty-five to decide to become a dentist faces many more difficulties than the person who began to prepare in junior high school. In fact, some children have a goal in mind as young as seven or eight years old, and even at that young age begin to concentrate and excel academically. At least, the possibility of becoming a professional ought to enter the subconscious minds of minority children as soon as they are born. If a minority youngster has never seen or even heard of a minority dentist, it is remote indeed that he or she would get the idea of becoming a dentist regardless of how well suited he or she might be for the career. An invisible network and support system exists in any class or group of people, and this is certainly true of dentists. These connections are not available to minority young people if no minorities are represented within the group. By getting to know many professionals as a young-ster, a student is able to gain subtle bits of knowledge that will help in the career choice as well as in the career itself.

Third, it is believed that minority patients will be more likely to seek care from professionals of their own race. Unfortunately, there can be a barrier in the mind of either the patient or the doctor that can greatly hinder the delivery of health care. Distrust by either party usually results in the patient's not following the doctor's home-care advice, and the patient may not return for the necessary follow-up care or checkups. The doctor, although highly competent and conscientious clinically, may not even have recognized what was really happening on an interpersonal level with the patient. In fact, some minority persons refuse to be treated by white, male doctors and instead seek out home remedies or nontrained, illegal practitioners. With more and more minority dentists available to them, these patients may now procure treatment as soon as a problem is discerned; even better, they may be receptive to preventive dentistry when it is explained to them by another member of a minority group.

The fourth benefit is the location of dental offices closer to the neighborhoods where minorities are concentrated. Some dentists are afraid to set up offices in those neighbor-hoods, but a person who was born and raised there feels comfortable and may want to set up practice there. It is disconcerting for anyone to travel out of his or her environs, enter an unfamiliar office, and place him or herself in the hands of a total stranger. It is just as disconcerting for the doctor to treat a foreign patient who may not even speak the

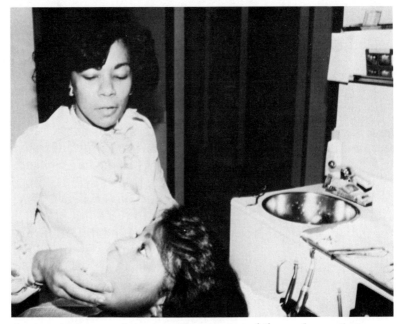

Dr. Joan Lanier, an endodontist, performs root canal therapy for a patient.

same language; it is downright unnerving for a doctor to treat a hostile patient of any race. Of course, the private doctor can order patients to leave his or her office or refuse to treat certain patients, but this does nothing to solve the problem of breaking down the walls between need for health care and its provision. When a minority dentist is available, it is natural that minority patients will seek him or her out. Then, if the patient has to be referred to a nonminority colleague, the patient will be able to trust this stranger, based upon the recommendation of the referring dentist.

Of course, a minority dentist can practice dentistry anywhere, and the presence of these well-educated, articulate families in previously all-white neighborhoods is dispelling and disarming racial prejudices. Change is slow, however, and minority dentists can still expect to face ignorance and bias from ill-informed and uneducated people. The less fortunate members of their own race may even show jealous contempt for that person's success. Various clubs and groups have been organized to give emotional support to minority dentists. To name just a few, there are the National Dental Association, an association of black dentists, the American Indian Doctors Association, and the Alpha Omega Fraternity, an association of Jewish dentists. These clubs offer social and educational programs as well as moral support.

Traditionally, women have not sought out a dental education in the U.S. In other regions, such as Eastern Europe and Russia, the majority of dentists are women. Why these sexual biases developed is a point of much speculation. The undeniable fact is that women are as capable of providing exceptional dentistry as men are.[1] Enrollment of female dental students increased more than ten times since 1970; in 1972, 40 female students graduated from dental schools in the U.S. In 1986 a quarter of freshman were women.[2] In 1989, 34.4 percent of first-year places in U.S. dental schools were filled by women; that represents 5,385 women in the entering class. Yet few teenage girls automatically answer that dentistry is their first career choice. The option may not have been presented to them, or they may not even have heard of a woman dentist. In Chapter IV, on educational requirements, it was mentioned that high school and college requirements for entering professional school should be well thought out in the teen years. Yet many women find they have been steered onto a track that locks them into traditional female jobs such as dental assistant and dental hygienist. Let me emphasize that there is virtually no degree of cross-over from one program to another. In fact, dental assisting or dental hygiene classes are not even considered acceptable as undergraduate requirements to enter dental school. Valuable time, money, and effort have been wasted when a young woman finds, at age twenty-five or thirty, that she is better suited to being a

[1] White, Mare V., D.D.S., "Dental Patients' Perceptions of Women Dentists." American Dental Association *Journal*, Vol. 105, pp. 223–230.
[2] American Dental Association Annual Report: Dental Education, 1989–1990.

dentist than an auxiliary. It is not impossible, and it has been done, but it is unlikely that a woman will return to college at that age to earn the minimum two or three years of credit to qualify for dental school. Where will she find the finances and time to pursue the career she has discovered she is best qualified to do? What if she has a husband and family to think about? Will they relocate to another city where the dental school she wishes to attend is located? If she had been able to weigh all the pros and cons as a teenager, she might have chosen dentistry to begin with, to her and society's benefit.

Women who find themselves sidetracked into an auxiliary role will enjoy considerably less power, control, autonomy, and money throughout their lives than those who made a conscious choice and effort to develop their potential in the teenage years. There may have been a time when male dentists resented women dentists, but as these males

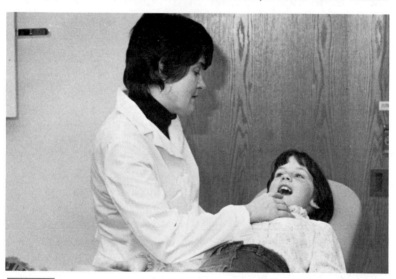

Dr. Sondra Gunn, an orthodontist, teaches at the University of Michigan and also provides orthodontic services at the Children's Aid Society in Detroit. She was a teacher before she decided to enter dentistry.

have daughters of their own and realize the sexual prejudices their daughters have to face, they are rethinking their
own biases. There is no reason to think women cannot
develop into outstanding practitioners in the dental profession, and there is no reason a young woman should not
consider entering the field.

The American Association of Women Dentists represents
many of the women dentists in the U.S. Most of the women
dentists are quite young, certainly younger than forty,
because there was a time not too long ago when class after
class of dentists graduated without even one female face in
the crowd. So the sprinkling of women dentists throughout
the fabric of society is still sparse. Dentistry is changed by
the presence of women; in 1980, 17.5 percent of all active
female dentists reported that they treated patients less than
thirty hours per week, compared to 9.6 percent of active
male dentists. Higher proportions of female dentists than
male dentists are graduate students, with most women spe-
cializing in orthodontics or pedodontics. Higher proportions of female than male active dentists are dental school
faculty members or employees of local, state, and federal
government.[3] In the dental schools, the female faculty
members are at the lower rungs of the teaching positions
simply because female dentists have not been around long
enough to accumulate the years and publications it takes to
move from instructor to assistant professor to associate
professor to full professor.

Women can still expect to face some sexual bias, from old
and young male dentists, and it is a foolish girl who thinks
society is waiting to welcome her with open arms when she
obtains her dental degree. In fact, much of the prejudice a
woman dentist faces comes from other women, women who
may have never had to complete a difficult task and so do
not think another woman can capably handle exacting

---

[3]American Dental Association, "Distribution of Dentists, 1979."

situations. However, in a study in the August, 1982, American Dental Association *Journal* it was stated that *generally*, "female dentists are not perceived as less competent than male dentists, and, in fact, may be perceived more positively on those dimensions reflecting warmth and gentleness in patient care. Young women considering dentistry as a career need not worry about sacrificing their femininity in the process, at least as far as their patients' perceptions are concerned." This same study showed that combining family and career responsibilities may well present a challenge to the female dentist, but that patients expect that she will accomplish both and that her family will not present a barrier to her able practice of dentistry.

A larger and more troubling problem a woman dentist faces is shared by all professional women: our society does not recognize the career woman as part of the family structure and does not address the problems a family with two working parents has to face. Although many women are now in the workforce, the traditions, customs, laws, and perks in this country are set up to benefit the family in which two nondivorced parents are raising biological children, with the mother staying home all the time as the father goes off to a nine-to-five job.

Working parents are faced with a system that allows large tax-deductible expenditures for business lunches but only minimally deductible expenses for child care. Isn't it obvious to *any working parent* that adequate child care is more important than a business lunch? That clean clothes and nutritious meals for children are more important than a company car or a new company logo? The working parents will have 'o wait for the lumbering government to notice that things have changed from the grade-school-primer family of the early fifties, where Dick and Jane and Mommy wave as Daddy drives off to his important job. Perhaps when more women are elected to public office, the needs of all families will be met in this country. Then the needs of professional women will also be addressed.

Running a dental office can be exhausting, but running a household and raising children is also taxing. They are simply different types of exhaustion. Attention has to be paid to the fact that the woman who enters the working world may hold down two jobs, one at the office and the other when she gets home to the children and husband. A woman who puts herself in this situation may be hazarding her health, mental, physical, and spiritual. An equitable balance can be achieved whereby the professional woman, her husband, and her children can all be adequately cared for. A quiet, revolutionary division of labor is taking place in American homes with two working parents, but there are few role models to follow.

A young woman must realize that practicing dentistry and raising a family requires a very delicate equilibrium, calling upon very different skills. Within a short time she will have to do a 180-degree turnabout in her emotions and responses. From nine to five she has to maintain a rigid time schedule; at five she has to loosen up because home life requires a great deal of flexibility. At the office, the dentist has to exude confidence and authority to the patients and staff; she has to demand perfection. At home, she has to cooperate and understand and expect imperfection. There, she is the supportive wife. In the office, the auxiliaries fulfill this function for her, constantly reassuring the patients what a great dentist she is. At home, she may be a flirtatious seductress; there is no place for flirtation in any dental office—in fact, an air of definite professionalism has to be maintained by the entire staff at all times. In the home, she has to be an empathetic friend, always ready to forgive. At work, she should not become involved in the staff's private lives. She has to expect the staff to perform optimally and has to fire those who consistently do not. She has to expect and demand payment from insurance companies and patients. She has to deal with dental repairs and supplies and cannot back down in her expectations when her demands are not met. With her children, on the other hand, she has to be a nurturing parent, freely giving of her time and self upon demand. In the office, a certain amount of nurturing can help with child patients, but more often than not the dentist has to take command and direct the child patient. She cannot waver when the situation calls for immediate re-implantation of an avulsed permanent tooth for a screaming eight-year-old. When there is evidence of child abuse, she cannot kowtow to the parents; she has to act in the best interest of the child and her profession.

Where their own children are concerned, a father can be as good a provider of care as a mother—even better, in some cases. It is an unusual father who cannot rise to the task of providing daily care for his own children when faced with that responsibility. As far as running the household goes, many services may have to be purchased. The laundry can be sent out, a cook hired, and a baby-sitter or nursery school engaged. The money a man and woman earn together will have to be used for these items, even though they were seldom part of a family budget in the recent past; and it is a large portion of the household income that will go toward the purchase of these services. The private dentist does have the option of scheduling his or her own hours. It is not unusual for a parent of infants and toddlers to work part time during the childbearing and child-rearing years. This allow dentists to keep up their other skills and expertise and also to give ample time to the family. To a degree, family activities can be planned around the practice, and the practice can be planned around the family.

Throughout her schooling, the dentist is taught to be competitive and hard-charging and achievement-oriented. In focusing on her training, she necessarily becomes self-centered. After all, didn't her parents sacrifice to send her to school? Or society at large through establishing schools and scholarships? Or her church? All her young life, others have made it possible for her to be schooled, and she has been encouraged to ignore any and everyone to concentrate on *her* schoolwork. With a family, she is now called upon to ignore herself and to respond to everyone else's needs. In school, she is taught that if she studies hard enough and really tries, everything will turn out all right. With a family, she is going to find that even with all the hard work imaginable, there are times when not everything can turn out "right." In order to succeed in any profession, a young woman has to learn to "psych herself up." There is a constant level of tension that enables her to perform her best in school, music, sports, and the theater. In the childbearing and child-raising years, she has to erase this subconscious tension and act "instinctively" and "naturally." Perhaps

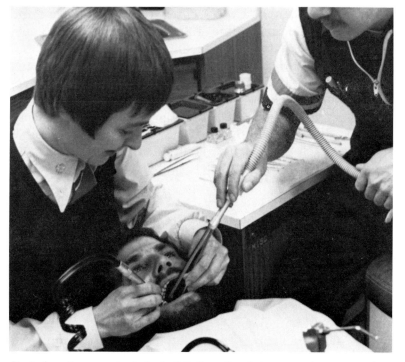

Dr. Barbara Bursaw, a dentist in the U.S. Coast Guard, does an amalgam preparation. She has traveled extensively in the Coast Guard, as far north as Alaska. In this photo, she is in Traverse City Air Station (William A. Strait Phtography).

there was a time when the bearing and rearing of children, the establishment of a family, was "instinctive and natural," but by the time a woman has gone through twenty-two years of schooling and a few years of practice, there may not be much instinct left. Then, just when she thought she had all the answers, she has to reexamine her life and priorities in order to try to create a happy balance between professional and family life. A wise young woman will explore all the equally important facets of her life as a dentist, wife, and mother before she finds herself in a crisis situation at the office or at home.

There is no reason for a woman to give up either career or family, but she has to realize that the balancing of both is difficult. She cannot expect either the profession or the family to be understanding if she herself does not understand what she is trying to accomplish, and why.

Talented men and women of all ages and colors and faiths are encouraged to choose dentistry and to guide the profession's future course, as well as the future course of society as a whole. If you think you can help the profession and society face the difficult questions ahead, by all means possible strive to reach your highest goals.

VII

When I was a girl growing up, there wasn't much thought given to the dentist. We all expected to lose our teeth eventually, and I did when I was forty-four. I couldn't believe how my life changed then; it became much more difficult to speak, laugh, and eat. My lips sank in. I bit my tongue constantly. It was awful, but I had no choice but to adjust. The dentist was very kind, and he helped me to adjust; he retired soon after. I did not realize that I should have my dentures checked once a year, and I even made the mistake of lining them myself.

Eventually they were such a mess that I could only keep them in my mouth for special occasions, for no more than two or three hours. Finally my daughter made an appointment with her dentist so that I could be refitted. Unfortunately, it was not that easy. I had damaged my ridges, and the dentist decided to refer me to a specialist because she did not think she could fit me properly.

I was pretty upset, but I knew something had to be done. The specialist, Dr. Baylor, was so kind that I immediately knew he could help me. He and an oral surgeon, Dr. West, presented several alternatives to me; they all involved surgery. I finally decided against implants and opted for the surgery that exposes more of the lower ridge by lowering the muscle attachments. There was extra, flabby tissue on the top that had to be trimmed away, also. The surgery was not pleasant, and it was a while before I was healed. Then Dr.

Baylor made a special set of dentures with a metal base in the bottom. I was in his office at least ten times. The dentures were such an improvement over what I had been trying to get along with; some of my woman friends accused me of having a face-lift because my lower face was so much fuller and less wrinkled with a proper set of dentures. I could actually chew again! But it's been so long since I had my real teeth that I cannot imagine what it must be like to eat without trying to hold these things in with my cheeks and tongue, to have something rooted in my head when I bite. If only I could go back in time and do it all over again!

But I am very glad to have seen Dr. Baylor and Dr. West. I know they did the best for me that they could. I will be certain to visit Dr. Baylor at least once a year to make sure these dentures fit right. I've got to protect what little ridge I do have left. And one thing is certain: I will do all that is within my power to get my grandchildren and great-grandchildren to see the dentist regularly!

This is Mrs. Gertrude Jenkins' story. She has just celebrated her 79th birthday and can be proud of the productive and full life she has had with her husband, five children, twenty grandchildren, and three great-grandchildren.

Chapter VII

Future Considerations in Dentistry

Technology has changed our world so remarkably and so quickly that we take for granted things our parents and grandparents never imagined. It is the same in dentistry. In a highly technical and scientific field, new ideas and innovations are always being presented to the dentist. Some of these developments are greatly beneficial to the profession, and others merely fizzle out. Nevertheless, many aspects of dentistry have not changed over the years, and one will never change: Because human nature and responses have not changed, dentistry will always be intensely people-oriented.

In the recent past plastics were introduced that revolutionized dental restorations. The new plastics, called *composites*, are harder, more lifelike, more accurate, and more durable than ever before. They are used to bond braces directly to a patient's teeth and to bond porcelain bridgework directly to the remaining natural teeth of selected patients. The latter procedure is so new that many practitioners still consider it experimental. Plastic and porcelain veneers are bonded to selected patients' anterior (front) teeth and greatly enhance appearance and function. Plastic implants, usually dacron-urethane, are used to strengthen weak mandibular and maxillary (jaw) bones and tempromandibular (jaw) joints, as well as other bones and joints throughout the body. The study of plastics is still relatively young, and greater use undoubtedly will be made of their unique properties in the dental field.

Improved metal products are being developed for use in the dental field. The amalgams (silver fillings) are far superior to past formulations. Research has also given dentistry new partial denture metals that are stronger and lighter than past alloys. Not long ago only a gold alloy was considered suitable for the basic structure of a crown or bridge, and the cost of the gold precluded its use for many patients. Now discoveries in metallurgy have allowed the use of nonprecious alloys as the basis for crown and bridge treatments. Dental implants are also being fabricated from the recently formulated metals.

A cosmetic development is the technique of cast glass ceramic restorations. Previously, porcelain was baked onto a metal jacket to provide a durable, esthetic restoration; however, the metal did not allow light to shine through the porcelain. With cast glass, an extremely durable, accurate restoration has been developed that allows light to shine through almost as in natural enamel. The restoration is then etched so that a special composite bonds it to the underlying tooth structure.

Computer software that records a tooth's shape, size, and bite, known as the CAD/CAM system, was developed in France and Switzerland. After preparing a cavity, the dentist hand-holds a wand that has a tiny camera on the end. The CAD/CAM scans the tooth and optically records its shape on a computer screen. The measurements are then transferred to a milling machine, which makes a gold or porcelain restoration. The fit, adaptation, and bite are as precise as the restorations currently being fabricated in the dental lab through many steps that involve three or four days. With CAD/CAM the dentist can cement the restoration permanently into place on the same day. This technology is also being used to generate periosteal implants, eliminating one day of surgery for certain implant patients.[1]

Implantology is bringing new hope to hundreds of patients who have lost their teeth. Past restorations were based on adherence to a patient's remaining tissues. Implants more closely replace what the patient has lost. New metal alloys and plastic compounds, even magnets, are placed directly in the jaw bone and are allowed to heal for six to eight months. Crowns, bridges, and even full dentures are then attached to the implants, providing a firmer foundation for function and speech. The appearance is very lifelike and pleasing.[2]

In recent years, a devastating disease called acquired immune deficiency syndrome (AIDS) has affected a growing number of the world population. Dentists play an important role in the early diagnosis of AIDS because many clinical signs of the disease show up in the mouth before the patient is aware he or she has it.

Dentists, as well as other health-care professionals, have to be careful not to contract the disease from patients and not to spread it to other patients or their families. There is no evidence that HIV (the AIDS virus) can be spread through contact with saliva or tears; the disease is spread through blood and semen. In dental and other medical practices there is repeated possibility of blood contact.

The Centers for Disease Control recommends that the following precautions be taken by all health-care personnel:

1. Rubber gloves are to be worn for all patients.
2. Protective eyewear is to be worn for all patients.
3. Masks are to be worn for all patients.

---

[1] Nash, Ross W., DDS, *Dentistry Today*; October, 1990.
[2] *Journal of the American Dental Association*, September 1990.

4. Gowns should be worn when blood contamination may take place.
5. Needles and scalpels and other "sharps" are to be disposed of in a puncture-resistant container.

In fact, the Occupational Safety and Health Administration has threatened to police health-care personnel and fine up to $10,000 those who fail to follow guidelines.

There is little doubt that third-party payers such as dental insurance companies and the government will continue to insure greater numbers of people. With this increase, more patients will be served by the profession, but there will also be more involvement and control over dentistry by non-dental forces. Many dentists believe this can only spell trouble for the patient as well as for the private practitioner. Nondental persons making decisions about patient care poses a serious dilemma to the profession. How can persons with no dental training make decisions that will affect patient care? The cornerstone of American dental and medical practice is being eroded: The patient and his or her doctor discuss the problem confidentially, and the patient decides what course to follow—including no treatment at all.

Critics of status-quo dentistry are quick to point out that the receiving of this fine care is based largely on ability to pay. They argue that the health professionals have not addressed the issue of poor and disadvantaged groups in our society who have not had and do not have access to health care. Many dental organizations have examined this need on a limited basis, but no comprehensive plan is offered by the dental profession to provide free, optimal care to all who seek it. The profession expects to be paid for its services and believes that any program providing care for underserved groups should evolve around payment through the private practice delivery system on a fee-for-service basis.

Someday national health insurance may be afforded to U.S. citizens. Whether or not dental care will be included in the initial package of such benefits has not been determined; for that matter, it may be many years before the U.S. develops a national health insurance program. Young people entering the profession must be aware of this, and perhaps they will bring with them a solution to the dilemma.

Recently some dental hygienists have demanded to be allowed to work outside dentists' supervision. Lawsuits have been filed in several states by hygienists who wish to establish their own "hygiene practice," separate from the dentist. A hygienist is licensed by the state, but it is generally agreed that the hygienist's two to four years of training limits his or her diagnostic ability. The hygienist cannot legally and is not trained to respond to dental emergencies and cannot write prescriptions. His or her ability to respond to a life-threatening situation that may arise in a dental setting is limited. Why do these hygienists want to establish separate practices? Many believe that they would make more money and that being required to work under a dentist's supervision limits their professional growth. The American Dental Hygienists Association is organized under the auspices of the American Dental Association, and the two groups are discussing the hygienists' as well as the dentists' concerns.

In the field of orthodontics a recent development is the use of "invisible" braces. The braces are bonded onto the teeth, on the tongue-side. The brackets and wires cannot be seen unless the patient tilts the head far back. This is a great advantage to adults whose careers limit the option of the unesthetic appearance of conventional braces. No more discomfort is reported with tongue-side braces than with regular braces; the tongue quickly forms calluses, and speech habits adjust rapidly.

Periodontal (gum) disease treatment relies on early detection. The FloridaProbe is an electronic, computer-assisted device that measures the health of the collar of gum around the teeth. Its accuracy of .1 millimeter is far more precise than the manual/visual metal probe currently in use. The FloridaProbe uses a microcomputer to generate a graph that displays pocket depth for a patient's entire mouth. The Pathotek is a culturing device that allows the dentist to determine whether gum crevices around the teeth exhibit active disease and what organisms are contributing to the tissue breakdown. The dentist is then able to "spot-treat" those sites and to prescribe specific medicines to eliminate the organisms.[3]

Lasers have been used in the medical and optical fields for many years. One drawback to use in the mouth is the nearness of hard and soft tissues. The hard tissues of teeth and bone generate heat when struck by a laser. The heat is high enough that the pulp of the tooth and the marrow spaces inside the bone may die. A laser for use in the mouth has been developed that solves the heat problem. This surgery does not require a scalpel; bleeding is considerably less; and the patient experiences much less discomfort and heals quickly.[4]

Genetic engineering now promises a vaccination that can be given to infants to prevent cavities for a lifetime.[5] Another idea is to create harmless bacteria similar to the bacteria that cause gum disease. When introduced into the mouth, the harmless bacteria replace the disease-causing organisms and the patient is "cured."[6]

Several scientists of the National Dental Research Insti-

---

[3] Laboratory Report, 1989, BioTechnica Diagnostics, Inc., 61 Moulton Street, Cambridge, MA 02138.

[4] *The New York Times*, July 14, 1990.

[5] *Dental Management*, December, 1990.

[6] Douglass, Chester W., DDS, and Furino, Antonio, PhD, Balancing dental service requirements and supplies; epidemiologic and demographic evidence, *Journal* of the American Dental Association, Vol. 121, November, 1990.

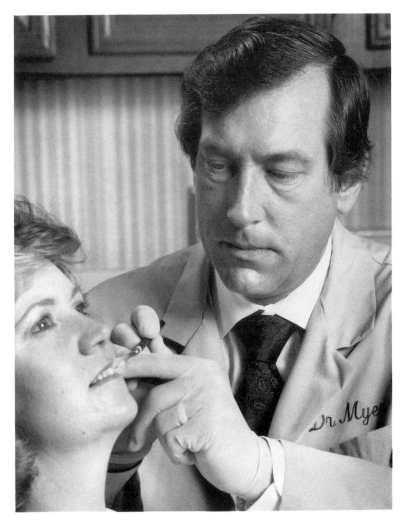

Terry D. Myers, DDS, co-inventor of the American Dental Laser, demonstrates use of the instrument on a patient. No anesthesia is required.

tutes are studying antiviral compounds, especially to alleviate the sores from Herpes Simplex I infections. Antibiotics specific to the infectious bacteria *Streptococcus mutans*, *Actinomyces viscosus*, and *Bacteriodes melanogenicus* are also being investigated and may well be beneficial elsewhere in the human body.

An important part of a patient's personality relies on appearance. The smile (or lack of one) is the dominant feature of the face. One aspect of an attractive smile is white and bright teeth. Several new medicaments are available that whiten and brighten teeth safely and effectively. Some of these agents are applied in the dental office; some are used at home under the dentist's instructions. Toothpastes are being formulated to lighten tooth color. These agents are especially beneficial for patients with tetracycline-stained teeth.[7]

Dentistry has always made great efforts in the area of pain control. In fact, the medical profession first learned about inhalation anesthesia in 1884 from a dentist who demonstrated the use of nitrous oxide to render a patient unconscious.

Dr. Silverston of the Oral Research Center at the University of Chicago is currently working on a dental pain suppressor similar to the "TENS" system. A headgear worn by the patient transmits 4 milliamps of electricity across the brain; the patient feels nothing. Within ten minutes the blood chemistry of the brain changes so that there is a 15 percent increase in seroton in and beta-endorphins, the body's natural pain suppressors. This allows almost all dental procedures to be performed without anesthesia. Some practitioners have begun to study accupucture and accupressure. It is too early to tell what effect this might have on general dentistry, but some young dentist some-

[7] Haywood, Van B., DDS, *Dental Management*, October 1990.

where may open a whole new vista of pain control for the entire medical profession.[8]

Another development is the sweetener Aspartame, formulated by the Searle Company under the trade name Nutra-Sweet. It was developed to reduce the caloric content of foods for obese people as well as for those such as diabetics who cannot use sucrose sugar. An added benefit is that the sweetener does not promote tooth decay. According to the manufacturer, Aspartame is not artificial but is actually a food, formulated by rearranging protein molecules.

Researchers are working on dynamic tomography, a technique of X-ray photography that can be used in the precise localization of tumors, foreign bodies, and fractures. The concept is also being applied to the tempromandibular joint (TMJ) to more fully understand its functioning or malfunctioning.

Dentistry is an exciting field that is changing every day. Research and dedication in the past have led to major changes in dental science, and the entire world has benefited. It is totally reasonable for all Americans to expect to keep a functioning dentition for their entire lives—even for ninety or a hundred years. There are talented young people considering dental careers who can make that possible. Brilliant young people like you can make a lasting contribution to mankind through the fascinating and challenging field of dentistry.

---

[8] Clinical Research Associates Newsletter, 1987, 3707 North Canyon Road, Provo, Utah 84604.

APPENDICES

Glossary

abscess Focus of injection that can occur anywhere in the body; in the mouth, abscesses occur in the soft tissue or the hard tissue. An abscess, commonly called a gumboil, is filled with pus, a mixture of dead bacteria, dead tissue cells, and white blood cells and other components of the blood that are trying to fight off the infection.

aesthetics The part of dentistry that deals with the appearance of a dental restoration. Usually it involves the front teeth and the matching of their restoration to the surrounding teeth in color, size, shape, and position.

AIDS Acquired immune deficiency syndrome, a disease caused by the HIV virus. The virus is transmitted by blood and semen; it enters the human body through breaks in the mucosa or skin, or directly into the bloodstream through contaminated needles or blood. The virus combines with the body's cells and destroys the immune system, which enables the body to fight off diseases or infections.

amalgam Physical result of mixing silver alloy and mercury. Pliable at first, amalgam hardens within twenty-four hours; it is used to restore back teeth.

associate Dentist who works in the office of an established dentist for a proportion of his or her own fees. The associate is not an employee of the established dentist, and so is responsible for his or her own taxes, insurance, and treatment plans.

avulsed   Referring to a tooth that is forcibly knocked out of its socket, usually by accident or trauma.

biopsy   Small sample of tissue surgically removed from the body in order for a pathologist to study its cells under a microscope.

bite plane   Also known as an occlusal guard, it is made of plastic and is prescribed for patients who grind their teeth.

Board Examinations   Series of tests given by a group of experts (a board) to determine if persons wishing to enter a profession are qualified to do so.

bonding   Dental materials that adhere directly to tooth structure.

bridge   Restorative structure used to replace one or more missing teeth. It is made of gold or nonprecious metal alloys; often, porcelain is baked onto the bridge to make it match the surrounding teeth.

calculus   Hard deposit that forms on teeth, fillings, braces, crowns, and dentures when plaque is not removed daily. The minerals in saliva and the fluids the patient drinks are trapped in the plaque and build up over time. The patient can remove the plaque by daily brushing, but only trained dental personnel can remove the calculus.

careers day   Day set aside at most dental schools for young people interested in dentistry to visit the facilities.

caries, carious process   Dissolution of tooth enamel caused by acid secreted by bacteria; the remaining soft material is usually brown; it is extremely weak and when removed, a cavity is the result.

cement   Material used to seat crowns, bridges, and orthodontic bands in a patient's mouth. It may be very strong, as for fixed bridgework, or weak, as for a temporary crown. Cement is also used under some restorations when the cavity is close to the nerve; it is intended to keep the tooth from being sensitive to cold and heat.

composite   Plastic filling material used in front teeth because it can be mixed to match the surrounding teeth.

crown   Covering for a tooth so weakened by caries or by trauma that it cannot hold a filling. Crowns can be made of gold, nonprecious metal, porcelain or porcelain baked onto metal, plastic, or stainless steel.

cyst   Fluid-filled sac lined by epithelial cells that may form inside the jawbone or in the soft tissues of the mouth.

degenerative   Pertaining to the breaking down of body structures and functions because of disease.

denturism   Making of dentures by persons who do not hold a DDS or DMD degree and who have not passed dental Board Examinations. Denturists treat patients in a variety of settings, usually in their home or at a dental lab.

Dental Aptitude Test (D.A.T.)   Test given to all applicants to U.S. dental schools. The test measures achievement and intelligence of the applicant relative to all other applicants.

dental assistant   Person who works under the direction of a dentist and assists the dentist. The dental assistant may have been trained in a formal program or by the dentist in his or her office. Some assistants are certified, which means they have passed certain tests and in some states may perform expanded duties.

dental hygienist, registered   Person who is qualified to clean teeth, take X rays, and promote oral hygiene.

dental technician   Person qualified to perform a variety of laboratory procedures according to a dentist's prescription. Most technicians work in commercial labs, but some are employed directly by a dentist. Some technicians are certified, which means they have passed certain tests and may perform an increased variety of procedures.

dentofacial   Referring to structures, hard and soft, that make up the face and the oral cavity.

diagnostician   Doctor who finds the cause of a patient's condition. All doctors are diagnosticians to a certain extent.

dry socket   Painful condition arising from loss of the blood clot in the socket that remains after a tooth extraction.

employee dentist   Dentist who works for other people for a salary or wage. Most employee dentists work in clinic situations, often with branches of government.

etiology   Underlying cause of disease.

extract   To remove a tooth from its socket by surgical means.

forensic dentistry   The aspect of dentistry that is suitable to be presented in a court of law to prove or disprove facts as evidenced by dental remains, restorations, bites, or X rays. Often, dental evidence is used to establish the identity of human remains.

franchisee   Person who has purchased the right to market dentistry under the name of a national corporation.

frenectomy   Oral surgical procedure whereby the muscle of the lip is detached from the jawbone so that the pull of the muscle does not separate nearby teeth or separate the gum from nearby teeth.

gold foil   Dental restoration that is formed directly in the tooth; small bits of pure gold foil are pressed into place in a sterilized, dry cavity.

gold inlay Dental restoration that replaces a missing part of a tooth with cast gold cemented into place.

handpiece Air-powered drill used by dentists to remove hard tissues (tooth structure) in the mouth.

hepatitis Highly contagious disease of the liver.

herpes Ulceration of the soft tissues of the mouth, usually a lip, caused by the *Herpes simplex* I virus.

implants Sterilized plastic or metal structures placed in a jaw to strengthen the jaw or to provide an anchor for a dental restoration.

immediate denture Denture placed the same day that teeth are extracted from the jaw.

infectious Pertaining to a condition in the body that can be passed to others by bacteria or a virus.

inflammation Reaction of the body to an infectious agent; swelling, redness, soreness, and a fever usually accompany inflammation.

lesion Any abnormality in body tissues.

license Legal right to perform certain tasks.

ligament Band of tough tissue holding bones together, holding bone to muscle, holding organs in place, or holding teeth in their sockets.

malocclusion Incorrect bite that results when the lower teeth do not meet the upper teeth properly.

mandible Lower jaw.

maxilla Upper jaw.

medicament Substance that cures, heals, or relieves pain.

National Boards   Series of tests given to applicants to determine if they have successfully completed a course of study.

neuromuscular   Pertaining to the structure and/or function of the nerves and their muscles as a unit.

neurologist   Medical doctor who specializes in the treatment of the brain and the nerves.

nitrous oxide (N_2O)   Analgesic gas used by dentists to relax patients.

occlusal adjustment   Grinding of teeth so that the upper teeth meet the lower teeth in an optimal manner.

operatory   Dentistry treatment rooms.

palate   Roof of the mouth. In the front of the mouth, the *hard palate* is supported by bone; in the back of the mouth, the *soft palate* is made up of muscle, connective tissue, and epithelium.

palsy   Paralysis and/or involuntary spasms of a muscle as a result of a disorder of the nervous system.

pathology   Study of diseases and abnormalities and their causes, usually involving the study of tissue under a microscope (biopsy).

periodontitis   Disease of the gums.

periradicular   Pertaining to tissues, cells, and fluids around the roots of the teeth.

plaque   Accumulation on teeth of bacteria, foodstuffs, and waste products.

post and core   Buildup and restoration of a tooth that is broken off at the gumline.

practitioner   A person who practices a profession.

primary provider   Practicing doctor who is the first person a patient consults. The primary provider may refer the patient to a hospital or a specialist.

pulp   Soft tissue inside a tooth, made up of blood vessels and nerves.

radiograph   X-ray photograph.

reciprocity   Recognition by one state of the legal validity of a dentistry license granted by another state.

saliva   Spit.

space maintenance   Orthodontic brace used when a primary (baby) tooth is lost early, to keep the teeth in position until the adult tooth erupts.

specialist   Doctor who makes a certain field his or her area of expertise; the doctor must study additional years in the specialty and pass a test in order to become a specialist.

Streptococcus mutans   Bacterium believed to be primarily responsible for caries.

suture   To sew tissues together in order to promote healing.

treatment plan   Before extensive dental work, a dentist outlines for the patient all steps, time, costs, and procedures involved.

third party   Person other than the patient who pays for health care; this might be an insurance company, the government, or the patient's employer.

tropism   Any response to a stimulus.

tempromandibular joint   Jaw joint.

visualization   Formation of a mental image of something not directly in sight.

Appendix **B**

Accredited Dental Schools

Dental schools that have approval, conditional approval, or provisional approval status are listed here. All programs have approval status except those designated with a cross (+) or an asterisk (*). A cross (+) indicates that the program has conditional approval status. An asterisk (*) indicates that the program has provisional approval status. The year appearing adjacent to the address of the institution identifies the year in which the next regularly scheduled on-site evaluation of the program(s) will be conducted. This identification does not preclude the commission from authorizing a site evaluation before the designated year.

Alabama
School of Dentistry
University of Alabama (1994)
1919 Seventh Ave S
Birmingham, 35294

California
School of Dentistry
Loma Linda University (1997)
24777 University Avenue
Loma Linda, 92350

School of Dentistry, University
   of California at Los Angeles
   (1990)
Center for the Health Sciences
Los Angeles, 90024

School of Dentistry, University
   of Southern California
   (1995)
University Park, MC 0641
Los Angeles, 90089-0641

School of Dentistry, University
   of California, San Francisco
   (1991)
513 Parnassus Ave, S-630
San Francisco, 94143

School of Dentistry
University of the Pacific (1994)
2155 Webster St
San Francisco, 94115

129

Colorado
School of Dentistry
University of Colorado
Medical Center (1995)
4200 E Ninth Ave, Box
   C-284
Denver, 80262

Connecticut
School of Dental Medicine
The University of
   Connecticut (1996)
263 Farmington Ave
Farmington, 06032

District of Columbia
School of Dentistry*
Georgetown University
3900 Reservoir Rd NW
Washington, 20007

College of Dentistry
Howard University (1987)
600 W Street NW
Washington, 20059

Florida
School of Dentistry
University of Florida (1995)
Box J-405, JHMHC
Gainesville, 32610

Georgia
School of Dentistry
Medical College of Georgia
1495 Laney Walker Blvd
Augusta, 30912-0200

Illinois
College of Dentistry
University of Illinois at
   Chicago (1992)
801 S Paulina St
Chicago, 60612

School of Dental Medicine
Southern Illinois University
   (1992)
2800 College Ave
Alton, 62002

Northwestern University
Dental School (1991)
240 E Huron St
Chicago, 60611

School of Dentistry
Loyola University of
   Chicago (1994)
2160 S First Ave
Maywood, 60153

Indiana
School of Dentistry
Indiana University (1992)
1121 W Michigan St
Indianapolis, 46202

Iowa
College of Dentistry
The University of Iowa
Dental Bldg
Iowa City, 52242

Kentucky
College of Dentistry
University of Kentucky
800 Rose St, Med Ctr
Lexington, 40536-0084

School of Dentistry
University of Louisville
Health Sciences Center
Louisville, 40292

Louisiana
School of Dentistry
Louisiana State University
  (1996)
1100 Florida Ave, Bldg 101
New Orleans, 70119

Maryland
Baltimore College of Dental
  Surgery
University of Maryland
666 W Baltimore St
Baltimore, 21201

Massachusetts
Harvard School of Dental
  Medicine
188 Longwood Ave
Boston, 02115

School of Dental Medicine
Tufts University (1995)
1 Kneeland St
Boston, 02111

School of Graduate
  Dentistry
Boston University Medical
  Center (1991)
100 E Newton St
Boston, 02118

Michigan
School of Dentistry
The University of Michigan
  (1997)
1234 Dental Building
Ann Arbor, 48109-1078

School of Dentistry
University of Detroit (1994)
2985 E Jefferson Ave
Detroit, 48207

Minnesota
School of Dentistry
University of Minnesota
(1992)
515 Delaware St, SE
Minneapolis, 55455

Mississippi
School of Dentistry
The University of
  Mississippi
Medical Center
2500 N State St
Jackson, 39216-4505

Missouri
School of Dentistry
University of Missouri-
  Kansas City
650 E 25th St
Kansas City, 64108

School of Dental Medicine*
Washington University
  (1992)
4559 Scott Ave
St. Louis, 63110

Nebraska
College of Dentistry
University of Nebraska,
  Medical Center (1994)
40th and Holdrege Streets
Lincoln, 68583-0740

School of Dental Science
Creighton University
2500 California St
Omaha, 68178

New Jersey
New Jersey Dental School
University of Medicine &
  Dentistry
100 Bergen St
Newark, 07103-2425

College of Dental Medicine*
Fairleigh Dickinson
  University (1991)
140 University Plaza Drive
Hackensack, 07601

New York
School of Dental Medicine
State University of New
  York at Buffalo
3435 Main St
Buffalo, 14214

School of Dental Medicine
State University of New
  York at Stony Brook
  (1993)
Rockland Hall
Stony Brook, 11794-8700

School of Dental & Oral
  Surgery
Columbia University
630 W 168th St
New York, 10032

College of Dentistry
New York University
325 E 24th St
New York, 10010

North Carolina
School of Dentistry
University of North
  Carolina
104 Brauer Hall, 211 H
Chapel Hill, 27514

Ohio
School of Dentistry
Case Western Reserve
  University (1996)
2123 Abington Rd
Cleveland, 44106

College of Dentistry
The Ohio State University
  (1993)
305 W 12th Ave
Columbus, 43210

Oklahoma
College of Dentistry
University of Oklahoma
 (1995)
Health Sciences Center
Oklahoma City, 73190

Oregon
School of Dentistry
The Oregon Health Sciences
 University (1996)
611 SW Campus Dr
Sam Jackson Park
Portland, 97201

Pennsylvania
School of Dental Medicine
University of Pennsylvania
 (1993)
4001 W Spruce St
Philadelphia, 19104-6003

School of Dentistry
Temple University
3223 N Broad St
Philadelphia, 19140

School of Dental Medicine
University of Pittsburgh
Rm C-333 Salk Hall
3501 Terrace St
Pittsburgh, 15261

Puerto Rico
School of Dentistry
University of Puerto Rico
 (1993)
GPO Box 5067
San Juan, 00936

South Carolina
College of Dental Medicine
Medical University of South
 Carolina (1997)
171 Ashley Ave
Charleston, 29425-2601

Tennessee
College of Dentistry
University of Tennessee
875 Union Ave
Memphis, 38163

School of Dentistry
Meharry Medical College
 (1993)
1005 18th Ave N
Nashville, 37208

Texas
Baylor College of Dentistry
3302 Gaston Ave
Dallas, 75246

Health Science Center-
 Dental Branch
The University of Texas
6516 John Freeman Ave
Houston, 77030

Dental School at San
 Antonio
The University of Texas
7703 Floyd Curl Dr
San Antonio, 78229

Virginia
School of Dentistry
Virginia Commonwealth
   University
Box 566-MCV Station
Richmond, 23298

Washington
School of Dentistry
University of Washington
   (1996)
Health Sciences Bldg, SC62
Seattle, 98195

West Virginia
+School of Dentistry
West Virginia University
   (1996)
Morgantown, 26506

Wisconsin
School of Dentistry
Marquette University (1993)
604 N 16th St
Milwaukee, 53233

Canada
Reciprocal agreement
between the Council on
Education of the Canadian
Dental Association and the
Commission on Dental
Accreditation of the
American Dental
Association was made to
recognize as accredited:

Faculty of Dentistry
University of Alberta
Dental Bldg
Edmonton, Alberta
T6G-2N8

Faculty of Dentistry
University of British
   Columbia
350-2194 Health Sciences
   Mall
Vancouver, British
   Columbia V6T-1W5

Faculty of Dentistry
Dalhousie University
5981 University Ave
Halifax, Nova Scotia
   B3H-3J5

School of Dental Medicine
Laval University
Ste-Foy, Quebec G1K-7P4

Faculty of Dentistry
University of Manitoba
780 Bannatyne Ave
Winnipeg, Manitoba
   R3E-0W3

Faculty of Dentistry
McGill University
740 Docteur Penfield
Montreal, Quebec H3A-1A4

Faculty of Dental Medicine
Universite de Montreal
2900 Edouard Montpetit
Montreal, Quebec H3C-3T9

ADA Principles of Ethics and Code of Professional Conduct

PRINCIPAL—Section 1

Service to the Public and Quality of Care. The dentist's primary obligation of service to the public shall include the delivery of quality care, competently and timely, within the bounds of the clinical circumstances presented by the patient. Quality of care shall be a primary consideration of the dental practitioner.

CODE OF PROFESSIONAL CONDUCT

1-A *Patient Selection*
   While dentists, in serving the public, may exercise reasonable discretion in selecting patients for their practices, dentists shall not refuse to accept patients into their practice or deny dental service to patients because of the patient's race, creed, color, sex or national origin.

1-B *Patient Records*
   Dentists are obliged to safeguard the confidentiality of patient records. Dentists shall maintain patient records in a manner consistent with the protection of the welfare of the patient. Upon request of a patient

or another dental practitioner, dentists shall provide any information that will be beneficial for the future treatment of that patient.

1-C *Community Service*
Since dentists have an obligation to use their skills, knowledge and experience for the improvement of the dental health of the public and are encouraged to be leaders in their community, dentists in such service shall conduct themselves in such a manner as to maintain or elevate the esteem of the profession.

1-D *Emergency Service*
Dentists shall be obliged to make reasonable arrangements for the emergency care of their patients of record.

Dentists shall be obliged when consulted in an emergency by patients not of record to make reasonable arrangements for emergency care. If treatment is provided, the dentist, upon completion of such treatment, is obliged to return the patient to his or her regular dentist unless the patient expressly reveals a different preference.

1-E *Consultation and Referral*
Dentists shall be obliged to seek consultation, if possible, whenever the welfare of patients will be safeguarded or advanced by utilizing those who have special skills, knowledge and experience.

When patients visit or are referred to specialists or consulting dentists for consultation:

1. The specialists or consulting dentists upon completion of their care shall return the patient, unless the patient expressly reveals a different preference, to the referring dentist, or if none, to the dentist of record for future care.

2. The specialist shall be obliged when there is no

referring dentist and upon a completion of their treatment to inform patients when there is a need for further dental care.

1-F *Use of Auxiliary Personnel*
Dentists shall be obliged to protect the health of their patient by only assigning to qualified auxiliaries those duties which can be legally delegated. Dentists shall be further obliged to prescribe and supervise the work of all auxiliary personnel working under their direction and control.

1-G *Justifiable Criticism*
Dentists shall be obliged to report to the appropriate reviewing agency as determined by the local component or constituent society instances of gross and continual faulty treatment by other dentists. Patients should be informed of their present oral health status without disparaging comment about prior services.

1-H *Expert Testimony*
Dentists may provide expert testimony when that testimony is essential to a just and fair disposition of a judicial or administrative action.

1-I *Rebate and Split Fees*
Dentists shall not accept or tender "rebates" or "split fees."

1-J *Representation of Care and Fees*
Dentists shall not represent the care being rendered to their patients or the fees being charged for providing such care in a false or misleading manner.

PRINCIPLE—Section 2

Education. The privilege of dentists to be accorded professional status rests primarily in the knowledge, skill and experience with which they serve their patients and society. All dentists, therefore, have the obligation of keeping their knowledge and skill current.

PRINCIPLE—Section 3

Government of a Profession. Every profession owes society the responsibility to regulate itself. Such regulation is achieved largely through the influence of the professional societies. All dentists, therefore, have the dual obligation of making themselves a part of a professional society and of observing its rules of ethics.

PRINCIPLE — Section 4

Research and Development. Dentists have the obligation of making the results and benefits of their investigative efforts available to all when they are useful in safeguarding or promoting the health of the public.

Code of Professional Conduct

4-A *Devices and Therapeutic Methods*
Except for formal investigative studies, dentists shall be obliged to prescribe, dispense or promote only those devices, drugs and other agents whose complete formulae are available to the dental profession. Dentists shall have the further obligation of not holding out as exclusive any device, agent, method or technique.

4-B *Patents and Copyrights*
Patents and copyrights may be secured by dentists provided that such patents and copyrights shall not be used to restrict research or practice.

PRINCIPLE—Section 5

Professional Announcement. In order to properly serve the public, dentists should represent themselves in a manner that contributes to the esteem of the profession. Dentists should not misrepresent their training and competence in any way that would be false or misleading in any material respect.*

5-A *Advertising*

Although any dentist may advertise, no dentist shall advertise or solicit patients in any form of communication in a manner that is false or misleading in any material respect.*

5-B *Name of Practice*

Since the name under which a dentist conducts his practice may be a factor in the selection process of the patient, the use of a trade name or any assumed name that is false or misleading in any material respect is unethical.

Use of the name of a dentist no longer actively associated with the practice may be continued for a period not to exceed one year.*

5-C *Announcement of Specialization and Limitation of Practice*

This Section and Section 5-D are designed to help the public make an informed selection between the practitioner who has completed an accredited program beyond the dental degree and a practitioner who has not completed such a program.

The special areas of dental practice approved by the American Dental Association and the designation for ethical specialty announcement and limitation of practice are: dental public health, endodontics, oral pathology, oral and maxillofacial surgery, orthodontics, pedodontics (dentistry for children), periodontics and prosthodontics.

Dentists who choose to announce specialization should use "specialist in" or "practice limited to" and shall limit their practice exclusively to the announced special area(s) of dental practice, provided at the time of the announcement such dentists have met in each approved specialty for which they announce the existing educational requirements and standards set forth by the American Dental Association

Dentists who use their eligibility to announce as specialists to make the public believe that specialty services rendered in the dental office are being rendered by qualified specialists when such is not the case are engaged in unethical conduct. The burden of responsibility is on specialists to avoid any inference that general practitioners who are associated with specialists are qualified to announce themselves as specialists.

General Standards. The following are included within the standards of the American Dental Association for determining what dentists have the education, experience and other appropriate requirements for announcing specialization and limitations of practice:

1. The special area(s) of dental practice and an appropriate certifying board must be approved by the American Dental Association.

2. Dentists who announce as specialists must have successfully completed an educational program accredited by the Commission on Dental Accreditation, two or more years in length, as specified by the Council on Dental Education or be diplomates of a nationally recognized certifying board. The scope of the individual specialist's practice shall be governed

by the educational standards for the specialty in which the specialist is announcing.

3. The practice carried on by dentists who announce as specialists shall be limited exclusively to the special area(s) of dental practice announced by the dentist.

Standards for Multiple-Specialty Announcements
Educational criteria for announcement by dentists in additional recognized specialty areas are the successful completion of an educational program accredited by the Commission on Dental Accreditation in each area for which the dentist wishes to announce.

Dentists who completed their advanced education in programs listed by the Council on Dental Education prior to the initiation of the accreditation process in 1967 and who are currently ethically announcing as specialists in a recognized area may announce in additional areas provided they are educationally qualified or are certified diplomates in each area for which they wish to announce. Documentation of successful completion of the educational program(s) must be submitted to the appropriate constituent society. The documentation must assure that the duration of the progam(s) is a minimum of two years except for oral and maxillofacial surgery which must have been a minimum of three years in duration.*

5-D *General Practitioner Announcement of Services*
General dentists who wish to announce the services available in their practices are permitted to announce the availability of those services so long as they avoid any communications that express or imply specialization. General dentists shall also state that the services are being provided by general dentists. No dentist shall announce available services in any way that would be false or misleading in any material respect.*

*Advertising, solicitation of patients or business, or other promotional activities by dentists or dental care delivery organizations shall not be considered unethical or improper, except for those promotional activities which are false or misleading in any material respect. Notwithstanding any ADA *Principles of Ethics and Code of Professional Conduct* or other standards of dentist conduct which may be differently worded, this shall be the sole standard for determining the ethical propriety of such promotional activities. Any provision of an ADA constituent or component society's code of ethics or other standard of dentist conduct relating to dentists' or dental care delivery organizations' advertising, solicitation, or other promotional activities which is worded differently from the above standard shall be deemed to be in conflict with the ADA *Principles of Ethics and Code of Professional Conduct.*

INTERPRETATION AND APPLICATION OF "PRINCIPLES OF ETHICS AND CODE OF PROFESSIONAL CONDUCT"

The preceding statements constitute the *Principles of Ethics and Code of Professional Conduct* of the American Dental Association. The purpose of the *Principles and Code* is to uphold and strengthen dentistry as a member of the learned professions. The constituent and component societies may adopt additional provisions or interpretations not in conflict with these *Principles of Ethics and Code of Professional Conduct* which would enable them to serve more faithfully the traditions, customs and desires of the members of these societies.

Problems involving questions of ethics should be solved at the local level within the broad boundaries established in these *Principles of Ethics and Code of Professional Conduct* and within the interpretation by the component and/or constituent society of their respective codes of ethics. If a satisfactory decision cannot be reached, the question should be referred on appeal to the constituent society and the Council on Bylaws and Judicial Affairs of the American Dental Association, as provided in Chapter XI of the *Bylaws* of the American Dental Association. Members found guilty of unethical conduct as prescribed in the American Dental Association *Code of Professional Conduct* or codes of ethics of the constituent and component societies are subject to the penalties set forth in Chapter XI of the American Dental Association *Bylaws.*

Appendix **D**

Organizations and Services

The Alpha Omega Foundation
267 Fifth Avenue
New York, NY 10016

American Association of Dental Schools
1625 Massachusetts Avenue, NW
Washington, DC 20036

American Association of Women Dentists
Suite 1636
211 East Chicago Avenue
Chicago, IL 60611

American Dental Association
211 East Chicago Avenue
Chicago, IL 60611

American Hospital Association
840 North Lake Shore Drive
Chicago, IL 60611

D.A.T. Preparation Manual
American Dental Association
211 East Chicago Avenue
Chicago, IL 60611

Public Health Service
Chief Dental Officer
5600 Fishers Lane
Rockville, Maryland, 20857

D.A.T. Sample Test
ARCO, INC.
219 Park Avenue South
New York, NY 10003

National Dental Association
Cecil Cook
5506 Connecticut Avenue NW
Suite 24
Washington, DC 20015

World Health Organization
Avenue Appia, 12-11
Geneva 27, Switzerland

NATIONAL SOURCES OF FINANCIAL AID

Department of Education Program.

On October 17, 1986, President Reagan signed into law "The Higher Education Amendments of 1986," Public Law 99–498. This legislation, also known as the Higher Education Act reauthorization, renews the authority of the Department of Education to administer federal programs of financial aid to students and institutions. The new law makes significant changes in the student aid programs of importance to dental students, such as increasing the borrowing limits under the loan programs and allowing consolidation of student loans. Listed below are the major programs authorized in the Higher Education Act of 1965, as amended.

Please Note: Not all dental schools participate in every program listed. Dental students may obtain federal funds only with the approval of dental school personnel. Therefore, it is essential for students to establish a working relationship with their schools' financial aid officers as soon as possible.

National Direct Student Loan (NDSL) Program.[1] P.L.99-498 renames NDSLs "Perkins Loans," after the late Representative Carl Perkins (D-KY), who was chairman of the House Committee on Education and Labor for over 30 years. Direct loans (using money paid by previous borrowers from the schools' "revolving funds") are available to low-income dental students, through the dental school financial aid office. Students may borrow up to $18,000 for graduate and professional study, including any amount borrowed under this program for undergraduate study. The interest rate is 5 percent. Repayment for new borrowers begins nine months after the student leaves school. No payments are required while the borrower is in school; during periods of up to three years for service in the Armed Forces, Peace Corps, VISTA, or a similar tax-exempt organization; while active in the U.S. Public Health Service; or while temporarily totally disabled. Further, deferments are allowed for up to two years to borrowers completing certain dental internships, including dental general practice residencies, and up to six months for parental leave. The new law allows partial cancellation of NDSL debt based on years of qualifying service under several circumstances aiding a national purpose, including work in the Peace Corps or VISTA. Further information about the NDSL program may be obtained from the financial aid officer at each dental school.

Guaranteed Student Loan (GSL) Program.[1] The Guaranteed Student Loan program allows students to borrow from private lenders to help finance their educational costs. The federal government subsidizes the interest for qualified students, and loans are guaranteed by state or private nonprofit agencies. To be eligible for GSLs, students must demonstrate need according to a need analysis system established by law. Qualified graduate and professional students may borrow what they need up to $7,500 per year. The aggregate total for the program is $54,750, which includes any GSLs borrowed as an undergraduate. The interest rate must be consistent on all GSLs; therefore, dental school borrowers who have had GSLs in prior years at 7 percent, and who still have outstanding balances, will pay 7 percent. Borrowers who have loans with interest of 9 percent will pay 9 percent on new GSLs, and those who borrowed at 8 percent will have new loans at 8 percent. Beginning July 1, 1988, interest on loans made to first-time borrowers will be 8 percent until the beginning of the fifth year of repayment, at which time it will increase to 10 percent. Borrowers are required to pay a 5 percent loan origination fee (LOF), which is deducted from the loan proceeds. New deferments are available to first-time borrowers beginning July 1987 for circumstances similar to those described for the NDSL program. An administrative fee also is assessed on each loan, equal to 3 percent of the principal amount of the loan.

SLS/PLUS Loans.[1] This program, designed to supplement funding made available under the Guaranteed Student Loan program, was created in 1981. The program is now available as "Supplemental Loans for Students" (SLS) to independent undergraduate and graduate and professional students, and "Loans for Parents." The annual borrowing limit has been raised to $4,000, up to an aggregate maximum of $20,000. As of July 1, 1987, the program will have a variable interest rate of the prevailing annual Treasury bill rate plus 3.75 percent, up to 12 percent. Borrowers who currently have supplemental loans at 12 percent or 14 percent may refinance their loans at the new rate for a one-time $100 fee. The government does not provide an interest subsidy for SLS/PLUS loans. All borrowers have the option to begin repayment of their loans within 60 days after the loans are made, or to have payment of the loan principal deferred, with the interest capitalized while they are in school or other approved deferral period.

Loan Consolidation.[1] The 1986 law creates a new loan consolidation program that will allow borrowers with a minimum of $5,000 outstanding in any combination of GSL, NDSL, SLS, and HPSL to consolidate their debts. The interest rate on the consolidated loan will be the greater of 9 percent or the weighted average of all the loans. Lenders may establish graduated and income-sensitive repayment schedules with payback extended up to 25 years, depending on the borrower's level of indebtedness. For loan totals of between $5,000 and $7,500, borrowers will have up to ten years to repay; for loan amounts between $7,500 and $10,000—with at least $5,000 of the debt in GSL and/or SLS—they will have up to 12 years; debt between $10,000 and $20,000, 15 years; between $20,000 and $45,000, 20 years; and over $45,000, 25 years. Dental students will be able to include "other" educational loans (such as HEAL) in determining the length of the repayment period; however, the amount of other loans used in the calculation cannot exceed the amount of the consolidated loan. In other words, to be eligible for the maximum repayment period, a borrower must have at least $22,500 in GSL, NDSL, HPSL or SLS, and $22,500 in other loans. Alternatively, a borrower could have a consolidated loan totaling $10,000, and $35,000 in HEAL and other loans, but the repayment period on the consolidated loan would only be 15 years. The consolidated plan restricts the allowable deferments to periods of full-time study, unemployment, and disability. Thus, students are advised to seek assistance—lenders are required by law to inform borrowers of all the deferment and repayment options available to them—to obtain maximum benefit of the deferments for which they qualify. The Higher Education Act also created a program that allows graduates who have borrowed under the HEAL program to combine these payments with their consolidated loans. This Combined Payment Plan will be especially helpful to those students who have borrowed HEAL loans from more than one lender. Students should discuss additional details of this program with the financial aid officer at each school or with their lender(s).

College Work/Study Program.[1] This program provides jobs for students who are enrolled at least half-time and who have financial need and must earn a part of their educational expenses. (Because of the rigorous academic demands of dental school, some schools do not participate in this program.) A participating educational institution arranges jobs on or off campus with a public or private nonprofit agency such as a hospital. In arranging a job and determining the number of hours a student may work (up to 40 hours a week), the financial aid officer considers the student's financial need, class schedule, health, and academic progress. The hourly wage depends on the job and the student's qualifications, but is usually at least equal to the current minimum wage. Further information may be obtained from the financial aid officer of each dental school.

Department of Health and Human Services Programs

The Department of Health and Human Services administers the financial assistance programs described below. Dental students are advised to consult their financial aid officers, who will have up-to-date knowledge about how to apply for each of these programs.

Health Professions Student Loan (HPSL) Programs.[2] Low-income dental students are eligible to apply for HPSL loans directly from their dental schools. This federal program has been in existence for over 20 years. Institutions make the loans from their "revolving funds," which are replenished with amounts repaid from former borrowers. The loans carry an interest rate of 9 percent and may be made for as much as the cost of tuition plus $2,500 per year. Loans are repayable over a ten-year period, which begins one year after the student ceases to pursue full-time study at a dental school; however, deferments on repayment of the loan principal of up to three years are allowed for service as a member of the uniformed services or the Peace Corps or for advanced professional training. Further information may be obtained by contacting the financial aid officer of the dental school.

Health Education Assistance Loan (HEAL) Program.[2] Under this program, participating lenders, financial or credit institutions, dental schools, state agencies, or pension funds make market rate loans to health professions students. They are generally considered "loans of last resort" because there is no interest subsidy, no maximum interest rate, and students pay an insurance fee equal to 8 percent of the loan amount to cover the costs of the program. The annual borrowing limit for HEAL is $20,000, up to an aggregate total of $80,000. However, dental students may not borrow amounts exceeding their cost of education minus their available resources. The principal is repayable over a ten- to 25-year period, starting nine to 12 months after completion of training. Repayment of principal is not required during periods of up to four years of internship or residency training and up to three years of service in the Armed Forces, National Health Service Corps, Peace Corps, or VISTA. Interest payments also may be deferred while a student is in training. The interest rate is determined by the 91-day Treasury bill note for the previous quarter plus 3 percent. Thus, the HEAL interest rate usually varies every calendar quarter throughout the life of the loan.

Scholarships for First-Year Students of Exceptional Financial Need (EFN).[2] A program of federal scholarships for dental students of "exceptional financial need" is currently available. The scholarships are limited to first-year students and cover the costs of tuition, books, laboratory expenses, and other reasonable educational expenses. In addition, recipients currently receive a monthly stipend of $400 for 12 months, beginning with the first month of the school year. These scholarships are available through the dental school; further information may be obtained by contacting the financial aid officer.

Financial Assistance for Disadvantaged Health Professions Students.[2] A new program, similar to EFN, provides exceptionally needy dental, medical, and osteopathic medical students with stipend support of up to $10,000 per year. These grants are available to health professions students in any year of study.

Southern Regional Education Board (SREB).[3] Students in certain health professions who are residents of Alabama, Arkansas, Georgia, Mississippi, North Carolina, or Tennessee may apply for aid from the Southern Regional Education Board contract program. These participating states pay a supplementary fee to the dental school, thereby reducing the student's tuition cost. A certificate of eligibility is required from the participating state that nominates the student. For further information contact: Student Contract Program, Southern Regional Education Board, 592 Tenth Street, N.W., Atlanta, Georgia 30318, (404) 875-9211.

Western Interstate Commission for Higher Education (WICHE).[3] Students who are residents of western states without dental schools may apply to the WICHE Professional Student Exchange program. All western dental schools participate as cooperating schools in the exchange programs. The home state pays a support fee to the dental school to help meet the cost of dental education. The student pays resident tuition in a public dental school or approximately one-third of the tuition in a private school. The "sending" states are Alaska, Arizona, Hawaii, Montana, Nevada, New Mexico, North Dakota, and Wyoming. Applicants should contact WICHE for information concerning the exchange program by *August* of the year *preced-*

ing admission so that they can meet the deadline for certification by their home state, which is October 15 of the year preceding admission. For further information, contact:

Director, Student Exchange Programs
Western Interstate Commission for Higher Education
P.O. Drawer P
Boulder, Colorado 80301-9752
Telephone: (303) 497-0210

United Student Aid Funds. United Student Aid Funds is a not-for-profit corporation which guarantees loans for students who are unable to secure a guaranteed student loan or an auxiliary loan in their home state. The terms of the GSL and PLUS/SLS loans are the same as for the federally administered programs described above. For information about these or other student loan programs, contact:

Loan Information
U.S.A. Funds
P.O. Box 50827-MC 5702
Indianapolis, Indiana 46250
Telephone: (800) LOAN-USA
(800) 382-4506 in Indiana

American Fund for Dental Health (AFDH) Minority Scholarship Program. This program was established by the AFDH in 1968. More than 500 scholarships have been awarded to minority students since that time.

Scholarships are awarded for the first year of dental school, up to a maximum of $2,000. Students awarded a scholarship for their first year may apply for renewal for their second year. Applicants must be U.S. citizens, have been accepted by an accredited dental school, and be a member of an underrepresented minority in the dental profession. These have been determined to be American Indians, black Americans, Mexican Americans, and Puerto Ricans.

Interested students must apply by May 1 *prior* to the first year of dental school. Scholarship awards are based on a student's academic record, financial need, and character references. To apply, contact:

Director of Programs
American Fund for Dental Health
211 East Chicago Avenue
Chicago, Illinois 60611
Telephone: (312) 787-6270

Canadian Fund for Dental Education. Canadian students interested in obtaining information concerning scholarships and loans available to them should contact:

Canadian Fund for Dental Education
1815 Alta Vista Drive
Ottawa, Ontario, Canada K1G 3Y6

----

[1]Further information concerning these federal loan programs may be obtained by contacting: United States Department of Education, Federal Student Aid Programs, P.O. Box 84, Washington, D.C. 20044, Telephone: (301) 984-4070.
[2]These programs are subject to congressional modification in 1987 and 1988.
[3]These programs are subject to modification by state legislatures.

Index

application to, 68-71
costs, 53
course load, 54-59
interview, 71-74
student impressions of, 60-63
women in, 101
denture, 24, 112
specialist, 19, 77
diagnosis, 19, 76, 113, 115
right to, 4
disease, infectious, 7-8, 17
doctor-patient relationship, 3, 17, 29,
83, 93, 99
drug abuse, 8, 27
dynamic tomography, 119

E
educational requirements, dental
school, 49-78
endodontics, 19, 79
English, 33, 49, 51
experience
clinical, 60
volunteer, 39, 50

F
family
dentist's, 20-22, 88, 98
woman dentist's, 104-108
financial aid, 53-54, 62-63
FloridaProbe, 116
forensic dentistry, 8
franchise, dental, 92

G
gays, 27, 28
gloves, rubber, 26, 27, 113
goggles, protective, 26, 115
goodwill, practice, 81, 82
government service, as dentist, 20,
81, 86
grade point average, 33, 50
gum disease, 6, 19, 95-96, 115-116

H
health, dental, 3, 19
health maintenance organization, 93

hemophiliac, 28
hepatitis, 7, 26
herpes, 7, 26, 118
hygienist, dental, 9, 52, 83, 87, 101,
115

I
implants, dental, 112, 113
income, dentist's, 22, 87
incorporation, of practice, 81, 85
infection, tooth, 7, 24
insurance
patient, 23, 114
liability, 28-29

L
laboratory technician, 9, 45, 52
language, foreign, 50
laser surgery, 116
liability, business, 17
licensure, 15, 38, 75

M
malocclusion, 19
malpractice suits, 28
mandibular bones, 7, 111
manual dexterity, 34, 40
mask, protective, 26, 113
mathematics, 33, 49, 51, 64
maxilla, 7, 111
minorities, in dentistry, 97-101
missionary, dental, 81, 93
moral obligations, 38

N
National Boards, 77
National Dental Association, 101
national health insurance, 115
National Dental Research Institute,
90, 116
North East Regional Board
(N.E.R.B.) examination, 76-77

O
Occupational Safety and Health
Administration, 114
operatory, 12
oral